TECHNICAL FOUNDATIONS
OF NEUROFEEDBACK

Technical Foundations of Neurofeedback provides, for the first time, an authoritative and complete account of the scientific and technical basis of EEG biofeedback. Beginning with the physiological origins of EEG rhythms, Collura describes the basis of measuring brain activity from the scalp and how brain rhythms reflect key brain regulatory processes. He then develops the theory as well as the practice of measuring, processing, and feeding back brain activity information for biofeedback training. Combining both a "top-down" and a "bottom-up" approach, Collura describes the core scientific principles, as well as current clinical experience and practical aspects of neurofeedback assessment and treatment therapy. Whether the reader has a technical need to understand neurofeedback, is a current or future neurofeedback practitioner, or only wants to understand the scientific basis of this important new field, this concise and authoritative book will be a key source of information.

Thomas F. Collura, PhD, QEEG-D, BCN, LPC, is the founder and president of BrainMaster Technologies, Inc., and director at the Brain Enrichment Center, Bedford, OH. He has held staff and teaching positions with AT&T Bell Laboratories, the Cleveland Clinic Department of Neurology, Case Western Reserve University, and Picker X-Ray (now Siemens Medical Systems). He has conducted research and development in the areas of brain evoked potentials, silicon integrated circuits, EEG brain mapping for epilepsy, quantitative EEG (QEEG), and neurofeedback. He has collaborated in the field of EEG with universities including the University of Illinois, Memphis State University, and Brown University. He is a past president of the International Society for Neurofeedback and Research (ISNR), and a past president of the EEG division of the Association for Applied Psychophysiology and Biofeedback (AAPB).

TECHNICAL FOUNDATIONS OF NEUROFEEDBACK

Thomas F. Collura

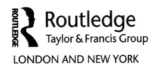

Routledge
Taylor & Francis Group

LONDON AND NEW YORK

First published 2014
by Routledge

2 Park Square, Milton Park, Abingdon, Oxfordshire OX14 4RN
711 Third Avenue, New York, NY 10017

Routledge is an imprint of the Taylor & Francis Group, an informa business

First issued in paperback 2017

Library of Congress Cataloging in Publication Data
    Collura, Thomas F., author.
    Technical foundations of neurofeedback/Thomas F. Collura.
    p. cm.
    Includes bibliographical references and index.
    (hardback: alk. paper)
    I. Title.
    [DNLM: 1. Neurofeedback. 2. Electroencephalography. WL 103.3]
    RC489.B53
    615.8'51—dc23
    2013008571

ISBN: 978-0-415-89901-7 (hbk)
ISBN: 978-1-138-05189-8 (pbk)

Typeset in Garamond 3
by Florence Production Ltd., Stoodleigh, Devon, UK

CONTENTS

ILLUSTRATIONS

Figures

Tables

Color Plates

INTRODUCTION

This book provides a survey of the basic technical underpinnings of neurofeedback, also known as EEG biofeedback. Our considerations will include biology, physics, electronics, biomedical signal analysis, computers, and learning. We will investigate the origin of the brain signals and the concepts surrounding the recording, processing, and feedback of these signals. This provides an understanding of where the signals come from, and how they are used in neurofeedback instrumentation. We will also explore the basic physiological mechanisms that underlie brain rhythms, as well as the changes in these rhythms that can occur in the course of neurofeedback training. These changes may be manifested in the ongoing measurements and also in changes in the behavior and self-reported thoughts and feelings of the trainee. These changes will then be put in a clinical context that should arm the practitioner with a solid technical foundation for practice or research.

Neurofeedback is based upon sound scientific principles that have been well established and documented through more than 80 years of basic and clinical research. This book will provide an overview of these principles, as well as references for readers who desire additional detail and support. Overall, the principles are rather simple. We are able to measure and identify brain states via recorded electrical activity, and we are further able to guide a trainee's brain to achieve and sustain desirable states, through straightforward instrumentation and computations. In the end, the brain is able to learn and adapt, and, in the presence of appropriate equipment and guidance, this learning and adaptation can have profound and beneficial effects. We have only begun to explore the capabilities of this simple, elegant, yet powerful approach to individual assessment, clinical intervention, and self-improvement.

At its core, neurofeedback embodies a process of neuronal self-regulation and re-education, leading the brain to find new and beneficial states and ways of processing information and feelings. However, it is by no means a "weak" intervention, and can be as efficacious as medication in many cases, and with fewer or no negative side effects. Applications are found with disorders as wide-ranging as anxiety, depression, ADD/ADHD, PTSD, alcoholism/addiction, and also autism, Asperger's, learning disorders, dyslexia, and epilepsy. With regard to clinical efficacy, the reader is directed toward excellent references, including Arns et al. (2009), Budzynski et al. (2005), Coben and Evans (2011), Kropotov (2009), and Larsen (2012). Neurofeedback is also used in nonclinical settings, including sports, performing arts, and academic proficiency, where its applications are designated variously as "peak performance," "mental fitness," and "optimal functioning" (Singer, 2004; Ros et al., 2006).

This material has grown out of a one-day workshop on this topic that has been taught by the author dozens of times in the past decade, often in conjunction with other established educators in the field. This workshop, which was first presented in 2001, grew from the demand of practitioners to understand the foundations of the science that lies beneath the clinical art of neurofeedback therapy. These practitioners have included, but have not been limited to, psychologists, psychiatrists, counselors, social workers, family therapists, chiropractors, nurses, and occupational therapists. This and related workshops have been presented to hundreds of practitioners under the sponsorship of the International Society for Neurofeedback and Research (ISNR), the Association for Applied Psychophysiology and Biofeedback (AAPB), and various regional biofeedback societies, as well as BrainMaster Technologies, Inc. and Stress Therapy Solutions, both of Bedford, Ohio. The result of the continual feedback and revision is that there now exists enough material to easily cover a week of instruction, while maintaining a focus on scientific and technical principles. As a solution to the problem of what to do with all the material that cannot fit into a one-day course, this text compiles and develops this material into a cohesive treatment.

It is hoped that newcomers and seasoned veterans alike will find this material useful, relevant, and interesting. As a complete read, it can provide instruction suitable for self-education, or even as a course text. As a reference, it contains details and clarification of many key principles that can be used as needed to answer specific questions. Overall, the intent has been to place neurofeedback on an objective and scientific framework so that it can be understood, practiced, and accepted as an evidence-based procedure.

The potential of neurofeedback as a therapeutic and as an agent for change has only begun to be realized. Much like the "barnstormers" who innovated aviation, or the "hackers" who pioneered early computing, the neurofeedback community of the last several decades has been characterized by devoted, creative, and open-minded individuals who refused to by stifled by convention. It should be noted that various matters of the art of practicing neurofeedback, the design of equipment, or the conduct of sessions are based upon field experience, and may not have cited references in the literature. They are provided here to reflect the state of the art, not as authoritative requirements.

1

OVERVIEW

Definition of Neurofeedback

Neurofeedback is a form of biofeedback training that uses the EEG (electroencephalogram), also known as the "brainwave," as the signal used to control feedback. Sensors applied to the trainee's scalp record the brainwaves, which are converted into feedback signals by a human/machine interface using a computer and software. By using visual, sound, or tactile feedback to produce learning in the brain, its primary use has been to improve brain relaxation through increasing alpha waves or related rhythms. A variety of additional benefits, derived from the improved ability of the CNS (central nervous system) to modulate the concentration/relaxation cycle and brain connectivity, may also be obtained.

In summary, neurofeedback consists of the following key elements:

- production of the EEG by the brain;
- recording of the EEG using suitable instrumentation;
- digitizing of the EEG into computer form;
- computation of EEG characteristics (signal processing);
- production and presentation of feedback (visual, auditory, tactile, etc.); and
- resulting learning by the brain, leading to physiological change.

This book will describe each of these processes in detail, and will thus encompass the areas of neurophysiology, biomedical engineering, digital signal processing, computer technology, and clinical therapeutics. In this chapter, we will provide an overview of the above concepts and present an integrated view of the process of neurofeedback.

It is important at the outset to distinguish neurofeedback from conventional EEG, and also from quantitative EEG (QEEG). Although these areas are related, they are by no means the same. Electroencephalography (EEG) is a technique by which the brain's electrical activity is recorded by the use of sensors placed on the scalp, and sensitive amplifiers. The EEG was first recorded by the German psychiatrist Hans Berger in 1932, and has become an accepted clinical tool for neurologists and psychiatrists. Generally, EEG is analyzed by visually inspecting the waveforms, often using a variety of montages. Neurologists are able to identify abnormalities, including epilepsy, head injuries, stroke, and other disease conditions, using the EEG. A clinical EEG practitioner in the medical profession must first be a neurologist or psychiatrist and complete an additional two-year residency and board certification in clinical neurophysiology, sleep disorders, epilepsy, or a related field to be eligible to read and interpret clinical EEGs.

Quantitative EEG (QEEG) is a technique in which EEG recordings are computer-analyzed to produce numbers referred to as "metrics" (e.g. amplitude or power, ratios, coherence, phase, etc.) used to guide decision-making and therapeutic planning. QEEG can also be used to monitor and assess treatment progress. QEEG data typically consist of raw numbers, statistics generally in the form of z-scores, and/or topographic or connectivity maps. QEEG systems currently lack strong standardization, and a wide range of methods and achievable results exist in the field. Although QEEG uses computer software to produce results, an understanding of basic EEG, and the ability to read and understand raw EEG waveforms, is required in order to competently practice QEEG. Generally, a specialist (e.g. a board-certified MD, PhD, QEEG-T, or QEEG-D) is consulted to read and interpret QEEG data and produce reports and treatment recommendations, unless the practitioner has appropriate experience and credentials.

Despite the fact that EEG, QEEG, and neurofeedback all make use of the same signal, they are based upon different sets of assumptions and clinical purposes. It turns out that a good understanding of both conventional EEG and of QEEG is important for the effective use of neurofeedback. In particular, in the areas of assessment and progress monitoring, a grasp of what a clinical neurophysiologist would think of the EEG, as well as what a QEEG practitioner would see, are both helpful in planning and evaluating neurofeedback interventions.

In contrast to clinical EEG and QEEG, neurofeedback can be ethically practiced by a wide range of practitioners with various backgrounds. Neurofeedback is not a "quick cure" or a "one-size-fits-all" intervention guaranteed to fix all ills. Rather, it is an evidence-based adjunctive to existing forms of treatment, and can be used by any practitioner who has reasonable training and is working within his or her own individual scope of practice. Therefore, psychologists, counselors, social workers, occupational therapists, language therapists, educators, and other professionals can incorporate neurofeedback into their work, or refer clients to neurofeedback therapists. Neurofeedback is best used when it takes advantage of brain plasticity to support and reinforce clinical goals in a manner consistent with evidence-based practice. In this regard, neurofeedback is on a par with other interventions such as psychotherapy, eye movement desensitization and reprocessing (EMDR), hypnotherapy, cognitive-behavioral therapy, and a host of other interventions targeting brain plasticity and change. While there are various certifications available for neurofeedback practitioners, there is no strict educational or licensing requirement; practitioners must first and foremost work within their licensure and competence, and add neurofeedback as appropriate.

Figure 1.1 shows a conceptual view of neurofeedback. We focus our attention in this analysis on brain events that represent specific patterns of neuronal activity. Some of these events are internalized in the form of thoughts that are perceived only by the individual as part of his or her internal world. Other brain events lead to external behaviors that are observed by others and also become part of the environment of the individual and are perceived as his or her own behavior. The normal pattern of brain activity is limited to this restricted space of awareness. The best that a clinician can do with regard to brain activity is to use a talk or

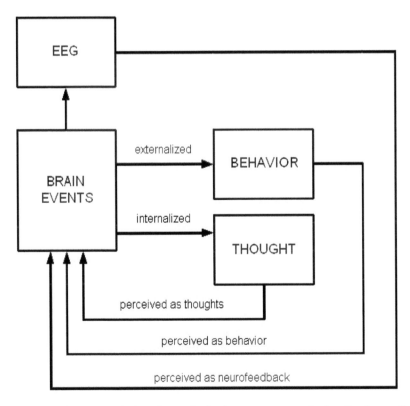

Figure 1.1 A conceptual view of neurofeedback as a component in the client's overall environment.

experiential/behavioral technique to alter the client's internal processing, or to use medications or stimulators to alter its function directly.

Table 1.1 presents a summary view of four of the major modalities available to the mental health practitioner. For each method, we look at whether it is based on learning, or on altering the brain, whether it has a strong biological basis. Specificity refers to whether the method can target specific brain locations or processes. Directedness indicates whether the intervention can be steered or directed, or is simply administered the same way for all clients. While there is room for opinion in this analysis, the general conclusion is that neurofeedback has the potential to be unique as a learning technique that is noninvasive yet biologically based, with high specificity and directedness in its ability to influence brain function.

Summary of Major Mental Health Interventions and their Properties

Neurofeedback introduces an entirely new facet to the experience of the brain events. With neurofeedback, an individual becomes aware of certain of his or her own brain events, and these then enter consciousness in the form of the neurofeedback experience. This is more than a mere therapeutic trick. It introduces an element of voluntary, as well as involuntary, control to critical aspects that have been hidden and now become part of the client's

Table 1.1 Options for mental health interventions

Modality	Method	Invasive	Biological basis	Specificity	Directedness
Talk/behavioral Therapy	Learning (various)	No	Moderate (when neuroscience-driven)	Moderate (cognitive/ emotional)	High (can focus on issue or problem)
Pharmaceutical	Altering (chemistry)	Yes	High (chemical change)	Moderate (neurotrans-mitters)	Low (widely distributed in brain, side effects and abreactions can occur)
Stimulation	Altering (electrical)	Yes	High (electrical conduction)	Moderate (location on head)	Moderate (polarity, location)
Neurofeedback	Learning (operant)	No	High (EEG and learning process)	High (site-specific or LORETA)	High (wide range of protocols, settings, sites)

decision-making repertoire. As we shall see, neurofeedback can be configured in many different ways, so that the external manifestation of brain activity that appears in the computer display provides the potential for change. It is as if someone who had never seen a mirror was suddenly able to see himself or herself, and to modify his or her behavior and appearance based upon this new information.

Figure 1.2 shows the simplest possible block diagram of a computerized neurofeedback system. Essentially, all contemporary neurofeedback devices operate according to this plan. Significant differences exist between implementations relating to the details of the amplifier, computer software, display, etc. However, this basic approach is a common factor, regardless of the system designer or manner of use.

Figure 1.3 shows one possible embodiment of neurofeedback, in which two participants are provided with information in the form of the movement of toy cars on a track. As the participants achieve the target set of brainwave condition, their cars move faster, thus providing a simple and intuitive form of feedback.

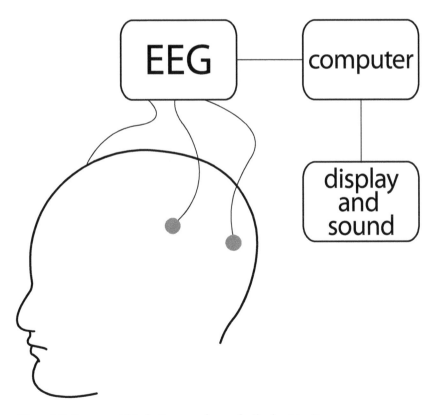

Figure 1.2 Conceptual block diagram of neurofeedback with client.

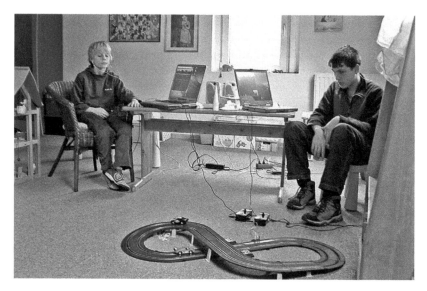

Figure 1.3 Two boys playing brain-controlled race cars as a form of neurofeedback.
Source: Photo courtesy of Dr. Doerte Klein

The following section provides, in a single narrative, the end-to-end picture of neurofeedback as it is viewed from a technical point of view.

Generation of the EEG

Pyramidal Cells in the Cerebral Cortex Produce Electrical Potentials

The EEG is a bioelectric potential that is recorded from the surface of the head, using appropriate electrodes and instrumentation. The human EEG was first recorded by Hans Berger in 1929, and within the following 10 years, all of the common brain rhythms had been observed and named, including delta, theta, alpha and beta waves. Measurable surface potentials (microvoltages) are produced by brain cells (neurons) in the upper layers of the cerebral cortex, which contains the outer information-processing layers of the brain, and which underlies essentially the entire scalp. The predominant EEG signals are produced by giant pyramidal cells, which are populous in layers II and IV, and are often oriented in a manner that encourages the production of measurable potentials. The cerebral cortex is divided into areas designated the frontal, parietal, occipital, and temporal lobes.

Based on the underlying physics, we understand that brain electrical sources are dipoles. An electrical dipole is a charged entity that has a positive "plus" side and an opposing negative "minus" side. For example, a battery immersed in a bath of salt water provides a good model of a dipole residing in a conducting medium. If electrodes are placed in the water bath, it is possible to measure the potential difference between any pair of points, thus measuring the voltage that would be analogous to an EEG measurement using two electrodes.

It is important to make two distinctions clear. The first is that the EEG is not there for any physiological reason, and does not reflect the brain's business in any direct sense. It is rather an "epiphenomenon" not unlike the heat coming from your computer, or the vibration on the hood of your car. It is a useful indicator of some aspects of brain function, but it is not a direct measure of information processing, such as a recording of action potentials might be. Second, even as it is detected, the EEG is not the "activity" of the brain. Rather, as shall be explained, the presence of a rhythm typically indicates that a region is idle and is in a neutral state. However, it may also indicate that region is "offline," or that it is "disconnected" from other regions. As tempting as it might be to make a value judgment that "large is good" or "smooth is better," no such simple distinctions can be made in EEG. As shall be explained, the bad news is that the neurofeedback practitioner really needs to learn a lot about the brain, how it works, and how EEG is generated. The good news is that all of this information is relevant, and neurofeedback is in fact a strongly evidence-based, brain-based therapeutic approach with extremely solid scientific foundations. In some cases, our understanding of neurofeedback is equal to, or superior to, our understanding of psychoactive medications, if one takes the time to look at the evidence.

EEG Amplitude Reflects Local Synchrony

Measurable EEG signals occur only when a population of cortical cells is excited (depolarized) in unison, providing a "consensus" potential, which is the sum of many small electrical potentials. If the cells behave independently, as they do when in an excited, active state, then the potential as viewed from the scalp are very small, due to the cancellation. Note that the measured potentials are actually epiphenomena, and are a byproduct of the normal activity of the brain. For example, consider the vibrations that can be sensed from the hood of a car. These are byproducts that can be used to diagnose and understand what is happening inside the car, but these are not fundamental to how the engine works.

Measured Rhythms Reflect Modulation in Activation and Inhibition

As a result of the previous considerations, it can be seen that the presence of a measurable EEG potential at any frequency reflects a measurable rhythm associated with local synchrony. Paradoxically, such synchrony may reflect the fact that a population of cells is actually not involved in active information processing, but is in an idling state. Many brain rhythms, in particular the alpha rhythm, are mediated by thalamo-cortical mechanisms that lead to the rhythmic interaction of different brain locations. In the course of its normal activity, the brain puts particular brain areas into a state of relative activation, or deactivation (inhibition). It is the modulation of these states that produces the characteristic waxing and waning that is visible in EEG recordings.

EEG Signals are Volume-Conducted throughout the Head

Exactly how do these brain potentials reach the scalp? Through a process that is known to physicists and biomedical engineers as volume conduction. The tiny neuronal dipoles produce circulating electrical currents that flow through the cerebral tissue and fluid, as it is a conducting medium comprised largely of salt water. Electrodes measure the surface potentials produced by this current flow, and are thus able to "see" the internal dipoles, by virtue of the surface potentials that are produced. As a result of this process, the electrodes will preferentially record from generators that are near the electrodes, between the electrodes, and oriented in parallel to a line connecting the electrodes.

In addition to neuronal electrical signals, other signals can be volume-conducted through the head. These include the electrical aspects of eye function and movement, muscle activity, and even the heart. The entire body, including the head, is more than 80 percent salt water, and this is a good conductor of electrical potentials. Therefore, when any EEG signal is measured, there will invariably be some amount of other signals, derived from other physiological sources.

Again, it should be kept in mind that volume-conduction is not a mechanism by which the brain does its "business." Rather, as a byproduct of normal cellular activity, electrical potentials are created, and these travel around the head by simple, passive circulation of electrical currents through the salt water that predominates in the brain. By measuring these signals, we are eavesdropping on a byproduct of brain activity, and using it as a valuable signal, for purposes of feedback, conditioning, and adaptation.

Measurement of the EEG

Sensors are Placed on the Head

EEG electrodes consist of metallic sensors that are placed on the head or on the ears. They make a direct connection to the skin. This direct contact is often referred to as "ohmic" or "galvanic," because there is physical contact with the body. In simple terms, the electrodes are sensing an electrical potential directly from the skin. Because the outer layers of the skin are typically poor conductors (good insulators), it is good practice to prepare the skin surface before applying electrodes. This preparation generally consists of a step of cleaning with an abrasive gel, followed by the application of the electrode, using a conductive paste, gel, or liquid.

The electrolyte is extremely important, as electrical charges are not able to move from a biological tissue directly into a metal. An intermediate electrolyte layer that contains an ionic conducting medium is required. Typical electrolytes contain chloride in an ionic form in conjunction with sodium or potassium, producing a conductive medium that can exchange charge carriers with both the skin and with the metal substrate of the electrodes.

Electrodes may be of a variety of materials. The most common are gold, silver, and tin. When a sensor is applied to the head, it will have a characteristic electrode impedance, which can be measured using an impedance meter. Typically, impedances should be below 10 kiloohms per pair of electrodes.

The electrodes are connected to *lead wires* that connect to the amplifier. The electrical potentials measured by the electrodes are conducted down the lead wires, to the amplifier inputs, where they are amplified. No appreciable electrical energy is taken from, or put into, the trainee's head. The US Food and Drug Administration (FDA), as well as industry standards bodies such as the Institute of Electrical and Electronics Engineers (IEEE), the Association for the Advancement of Medical Instrumentation (AAMI), and the International Standards Organization (ISO), have established the maximum allowable levels of any possible electrical "interference," and all legally marketed EEG systems must comply with these regulations through certified testing. This ensures that EEG equipment is noise-free and noninvasive. The amplification of EEG is an entirely passive process, in which a measurement of a microvoltage is accomplished using a very sensitive electronic device.

Differential Amplifiers are Used

EEG amplifiers are *differential amplifiers*. This means that they have two signal inputs, in addition to a "ground" connection. A differential amplifier measures the difference between two signals. The use of differential amplification is necessary in order to separate the EEG signal from other stray signals in the vicinity, including electrical interference due to other equipment. The two inputs are generally known as the *active* input and the *indifferent* or *reference* input. The signal recorded between one active input and its corresponding reference input is considered to be a single EEG channel, and produces a waveform corresponding to the changes in electrical potential between the pair.

9

Amplifier Quality: Input Impedance, Common Mode Rejection

EEG amplifiers have several attributes that are important to reliable and accurate recording. The most basic of these is the *input impedance*. This is a measure of how well the amplifier can measure electrical potential without drawing excessive current. Because the impedance of the sensors is not zero, it is necessary to have a high input impedance in order to accurately measure the potentials. The combination of the electrode impedance and the amplifier input impedance provides a voltage divider that reduces the measured potential by a fraction equal to the ratio of the impedances. It is not the actual reduction that is the problem, but it is the possible mismatch between individual electrodes that causes a problem. If the input impedance is very high, then the possible mismatch is very small. In the end, an amplifier with very high input impedance will provide a more noise-free and accurate signal than one with lower impedance. Typically, EEG amplifiers have input impedances of at least 1 gigohm (10^9 ohms), thus providing accurate signals with electrodes that have source impedances of up to 20 kiloohms or more. At the same time, electrode impedances should be kept below 10 kiloohms per pair to ensure good EEG recordings.

Signal Properties: Frequency, Amplitude

The frequency of a signal represents how fast the signal is moving. The amplitude represents how large the signal is. We refer to an EEG component as the signal that is associated with a particular band of frequencies, and is measured as a function of time. Strictly speaking, for example, an individual's "alpha" is not a frequency, but it is a signal that may occupy any of a range of frequencies. "10.0 Hz" is a frequency. "A brain signal that typically is centered near 10.0 Hz and is measured between 8 and 12 Hz" is one way of defining the alpha component. However, an even better definition would be "alpha is a rhythm that is maximal occipitally, increases when the eyes close, has a characteristic waxing and waning, and is typically between 8 and 12 cycles per second in adults."

Processing the EEG

Digitization: Sampling Rate, Resolution

In most modern EEG neurofeedback systems, the signal is first digitized, so that it can be processed using digital techniques. The signal is digitized by sampling it repetitively in time, and for each instant, producing a digital number that represents the instantaneous value of the signal waveform. It is necessary to digitize the signal with sufficient resolution in time and in voltage to represent it accurately, and to provide adequate feedback to the trainee.

The FFT is Like a "Prism"

The *FFT* or *Fast Fourier Transform* is a digital technique that takes a signal and produces estimates of the energy in a range of frequencies, broken into *bins*. The FFT is often used for assessment and display purposes because it provides a single, comprehensive view of all of the frequencies in the input. The output is generally viewed as a *spectral display*.

Mathematically, the Fourier transform, of which the FFT is one implementation, works by fitting the signal to a set of successive sine waves and seeing how much of each frequency exists in the signal. Thus, it surveys the signal across a range of frequencies and provides a value for each one. This is similar to the manner in which a prism takes white (or colored) light and breaks it into its components, each shown across a display, much like a white sheet of paper that has a rainbow projected upon it—in the same way that the spectrum provided by a prism can indicate the relative amounts of each color, by the intensity of its respective projection.

The Digital Filter is Like a Colored Lens

Digital filtering is a technique that uses computational techniques to process a signal, and to produce an output that consists of only selected frequencies. The output is thus a narrowband signal, or a filtered signal. This signal again has the properties of amplitude and frequency. Digital filtering is analogous to a colored glass that only lets certain wavelengths of light through, while reducing others. A digital filter passes certain EEG frequencies to make them visible, while reducing others.

Ultimately, the training signal is derived from the amplitude and frequency of the EEG. The amplitude is measured as the magnitude or size of the signal, which indicates the amplitude of the up and down excursions that comprise the oscillating waveform. Amplitude may be expressed as peak-to-peak microvolts, root-mean-square (RMS) microvolts, or as power, with units of microvolts squared.

A digital filter has several properties. The most important of these are the *center frequency* and the *bandwidth*. Alternatively, a filter can be specified by its upper and lower cutoff frequencies. These representations are equivalent, in that the center frequency is equal to the average of the upper and lower cutoff frequencies, and the bandwidth is equal to the difference between the cutoff frequencies. For example, a filter with cutoff frequencies of 8.0 and 12.0 Hz is equivalently described as one with a center frequency of 10.0 Hz and a bandwidth of 4.0 Hz.

Any filter is a real-world design, and has properties that are not ideal. Despite the flexibility and repeatability of digital filters, they still must conform to basic mathematic principles that cannot be violated. For example, no filter can completely remove signals that are outside of the passband. Rather, practical filters respond with a lower amplitude to such signals. The slope of the passband is a figure of merit for digital filters, and is indicated by the order of the filter.

The response time of a digital filter will depend on the type and order of the filter. Typically, any filter will require at least one cycle of a wave, in order to register the change. This built-in delay is unavoidable, and is a result of the mathematical properties of any filter. Therefore, the response time of a filter is a function of its bandwidth, and also the center frequency.

In order for a filter to be able to follow changes in component amplitude with time, it must be able to reflect these changes dynamically. The overall size of the signal, which is visible in the form of characteristic waxing and waning, is also referred to as the "envelope" of the signal. Such amplitude modulation produces sidebands that must be passed if the filter is to respond to changes. Typically, filters are set with a bandwidth of at least 3 Hz, and are often set wider. Extremely narrowband filters will exhibit resonance, and will be very slow to respond to changes in the input.

Another important aspect of signal processing at this level is the use of "tuning" parameters, such as damping factors, averaging windows, sustained reward criteria, refractory periods, and other modifications to the algorithms. In order to produce feedback that is aesthetic, smooth, and informative to the brain, it is often of value to introduce calculations that modify the time-response of the system in a useful way. Generally, if all of the basic signal processing elements are allowed to operate as fast as possible, feedback may be perceived as "jerky" or "too fast." The brain requires the training information to be appropriately timed and organized, to best suit the operant learning paradigm and to keep feedback pleasant and graceful. The importance of these factors, as well as their relevance to neurofeedback, is discussed in Chapters 4 and 5.

Coherence and Synchrony

In addition to training using amplitude-based measures, neurofeedback systems can also use connectivity-based measures. These include coherence, synchrony, and other related measures. A wide range of methods is available for measuring brain connectivity, and they each have unique qualities, strengths, and weaknesses. Some are found more useful in peak performance and mental fitness training, others with learning disabilities, dyslexia, epilepsy, and other applications. There is a long and complex history to EEG connectivity measurement and training, which is addressed in further detail in Chapter 6.

Thresholds and Protocols Set Decision Points

Regardless of the type of EEG metric used to produce feedback, it is generally necessary to introduce the concept of a "threshold," which is typically a value that an EEG metric must meet in order to achieve feedback. In its simplest form, it is a microvolt level that an EEG amplitude must be above or below in order to achieve a reward.

When a neurofeedback instrument is configured for use, it is necessary to define the signal aspects that will be used to produce (or inhibit) training rewards. One common method is to set thresholds, which are amplitude levels that are used for decision-making within the neurofeedback software. In conjunction with the thresholds, a protocol is used that defines which components are rewarded (or inhibited), as well as other details of the training process. For example, a system could be set with a threshold of 6.5 microvolts for theta, and an inhibit setting. This means that the feedback would only be forthcoming when theta is below a threshold of 6.5.

There are two basic ways to use an "inhibit." One is to use it to withhold rewards, if the component is above threshold. Thus, the component inhibits the reward feedback. Another method is to allow the feedback system to specifically produce reward sounds when the theta is below threshold. The difference in these methods lies in whether or not the theta going below threshold produces a feedback sound, or whether it allows a feedback sound that might be forthcoming due to other factors.

Data Storage Saves the Signal and the Results

It is generally desirable to review the results of neurofeedback training in order to assess the effectiveness of the training, to plan future trainings, and to debrief the client. The session data can be saved in several forms, which provide different types of information.

Statistics Provide for Informative Review and Decision-Making

In neurofeedback, it is important to ensure that the trainee is experiencing operant or other learning, and that anticipated changes in the EEG are observed. While it is possible to see improvement in trainees without significant change in the EEG, it is generally accepted that EEG changes are expected, and that outcomes are generally better, when EEG learning can be demonstrated. The simplest approach to this is simply to plot EEG values across time, either within a session, or across sessions. Neurofeedback systems generally provide some means for reviewing session data, and even exporting them to programs such as Excel, Access, Matlab, or other software packages for offline review and analysis.

How the EEG Information is Fed Back to the Trainee

Feedback is presented so as to provide the brain with information using visual, auditory, tactile, or even magnetic devices. There are a wide range of possible means to provide information to the brain, and even channels that are generally considered imperceptible, sub-threshold, or subliminal have the potential to be used in biofeedback and neurofeedback.

Generally, it is understood that the neurofeedback must have three key attributes. It must be rapid, it must be accurate, and it must be aesthetic (Hardt, 2001). Barry Sterman has stated that feedback must be correct, timely, and meaningful (Sterman, 2008). If any of these qualities are violated, the efficacy of the neurofeedback will be compromised. The key attribute of any feedback is that it is contingent on the EEG. This means that the feedback will be withheld under nominal conditions, but will be presented or altered when the target state is achieved.

Feedback may also use a sustained reward criterion to ensure that the brain is producing a sustained rhythm in order to receive a reward. This typically consists of the requirement that the target conditions are sustained for a predetermined time, for example ½ second, before a reward sound or point is issued.

Graphic/Text Displays Provide Visible Feedback

Visual displays generally fall into one of two categories, clinical or operator displays, and trainee ("game") displays. However, some displays are suitable for both purposes, and some neurofeedback systems do not make this distinction. A variety of methods are available for controlling visual feedback. These include stop-start, brightness modulation (bright/dim), contrast modulation (clear/faded), zoom in/out, or other changes that differentially obscure or enable the visual material to be seen.

Sounds Provide Audible Feedback

Auditory feedback can be either discrete or continuous. When discrete feedback is used, a single tone, such as a bell, click, or other simple sound, is used as the reward. There is generally a sustained reward criterion applied before the sound is heard, and a refractory period applied before another tone can be presented. In this model, sounds are typically heard every few seconds, and signal the successful achievement of the target state. Continuous feedback consists of sustained musical notes, chords, or even synthesized or recorded music, used as a continual indication of the EEG parameters. The trainee typically listens to the sound, and knows that as it becomes louder, he or she is achieving the training goals.

Tactile and Other Feedback

Other methods for feedback include tactile feedback, which uses perceptible vibrations, or "thumps," for feedback. This is particularly useful for the very young and the very old, or trainees who can benefit from the additional tactile component. Often, the feedback is provided with a stuffed animal or other device, which encourages the trainee to hold onto it and experience the feedback.

Another method of feedback is to use real-world devices, such as electric trains, toys, blimps, robots, race cars, or other external devices. These have the benefit of being intuitively clear to any user and simple to understand. They have the disadvantage of being generally costly and somewhat difficult to configure and operate, considering the many degrees of freedom and control required to keep a toy operating at a suitable speed and be responsive to the EEG conditions. One such device has been used on the BBC in a television program that used EEG-controlled model race cars as a competition between teams of competitors. While many expect this works simply as a brain-controlled device, in the manner of "you think go, and the car goes," the reality is actually the opposite. The car goes, and that tells you that your brain has achieved the desired state.

Another form of feedback may consist of minute amounts of energy, either in electrical (Ochs, 1994) or magnetic form (Ochs, 2006; Stahl and Collura, 2012). These mechanisms appear to have the potential to affect the brain through very slight shifts in phases, presumably through the modulation of transmembrane potentials at a very small scale.

Instructions to the Trainee

One of the most difficult things for neurofeedback practitioners to understand is what to tell the trainee, and what to expect the trainee to "do." Paradoxically, neurofeedback can work quite well in the absence of effort; the trainee can allow learning to occur without forcing it or attempting to perform a voluntary task. Neurofeedback is a means to allow the brain to learn a new state, or states, and to find its own way to implement the learning. While there is a volitional aspect to the learning, and while there may be subjective changes that are perceived, the trainee generally experiences the learning rather than making the learning occur. This is in contrast to some peripheral biofeedback techniques such as hand-warming, paced breathing, or heart-rate variability training, in which the trainee has specific and clear instructions, and "wills" the events to occur. No such coaching or effect is generally found effective in neurofeedback.

Generally, neurofeedback is an automatic process, and an important goal of trainee instructions is to allow the trainee's conscious brain to get "out of the way" and allow neurofeedback to proceed. Instructions such as "allow the sounds to come" or "relax and let yourself feel what it's like when you get a reward" may be used. The trainee needs primarily to use the points as a reward, to see his or her progress, and to let go and allow the brain to learn progressively, as the feedback trains the brain to go further in the desired directions.

If the trainee directs relaxed attention toward the feedback displays and sounds, and allows the natural process of learning to occur, the brain will spontaneously seek to satisfy the conditions of the feedback training, and to find the states that are being rewarded. As time goes by and training progresses, the trainee will often find it possible to go deeper and more consistently into the conditioned state and to maintain this state with less effort.

Although neurofeedback training is largely automatic and not under voluntary control, there is an important element of intention that consists of priming the brain to process rewards in a positive way. It is optimal if feedback is intrinsically appealing, novel, or desirable, so that the brain seeks feedback and hence fosters the targeted brain states.

What Happens in the Brain

Autoregulation

The process by which neurofeedback effects changes in the brain is one of auto-regulation, or self-regulation. Regardless of the trainee's intentions, the brain will seek to achieve states that provide rewards, however a reward is judged. For example, novelty is generally sought, unless it is unpleasant. Thus, if a system provides sound feedback under certain EEG conditions, there is a predisposition of any brain to seek novelty, and hence to learn to produce the specified EEG qualities.

Operant Conditioning

Operant conditioning (also known as "instrumental learning") takes place when an organism interacts with a system that provides rewards of some kind (displays, sounds, food, electrical stimulation, etc.) as a response to some behavior or state change produced by the trainee. Operant conditioning, or instrumental learning, is the process by which an organism learns to produce a particular behavior because it is rewarded. In the case of neurofeedback, the behavior is the production of particular brainwave patterns.

Each time the designated event occurs, the instrumentation provides a signal indicating this to the trainee. If the signal is perceived as desirable, then the brain will spontaneously learn to achieve the state that leads to the signal, over a long number of trials. Each trial becomes one more opportunity for the brain to review the moments preceding the reward, and to understand what has been done to get it. Note that this processing is not done at the conscious level, but is achieved by automatic mechanisms. These mechanisms may be "primed" by the trainee's desire to do well, or to make the sounds come. However, the conditioning process is an unconscious process, and is not under the same kind of voluntary control as a finger movement, for example. It is relevant to note that because neurofeedback is an operant learning technique, it cannot force the brain to enter any state or condition that it is not itself able to achieve on its own. Therefore, it can only reinforce and direct natural state transitions. This provides an element of safety, in that neurofeedback is generally incapable of "doing something bad" to a client. This element of safety is not achieved with medications or other more directive techniques, which do have the possibility of producing undesirable changes in the form of iatrogenic effects, also known as "side effects."

Operant Conditioning

The process by which an organism learns to produce a desired behavior (operant) as a result of being rewarded for that behavior. The target behavior is said to be "reinforced" by the reward. Operant learning theory was notably pioneered by Skinner (1938) and Miller (1967, 1969).

Intention to be Still, Focus, Relax

All brain rhythms are fundamentally those of relaxation. In particular, the SMR rhythm is connected with the brain's intention to be still. Whenever the body is still, and intends to remain still, the sensorimotor cortex is freed up to produce its idle waveform, which is SMR. Similarly, when the eyes are closed and the person is relaxed, alpha waves occur in the back of the head, associated with relaxation and background memory scanning.

Post-Reinforcement Synchronization

When the brain registers that a brief task has been accomplished, and that a reward has been registered (or is forthcoming), a signal known as post-reinforcement synchronization (PRS) can be observed. Furthermore, whenever the reward is withdrawn (or diluted, in the case of cats being fed milk), the PRS disappears, along with the disappearance of the behavior that previously led to rewards. This shows that the PRS is associated with the organism's sense of success, and comprises a mini-relaxation, or a signal to the brain to relax, and to subsequently get ready for the next trial.

Classical Conditioning and Other Mechanisms

In addition to operant conditioning, neurofeedback provides the opportunity for other learning mechanisms to become active. The processes that can take place during neurofeedback training include the following:

Neurofeedback Learning Mechanisms

- Classical conditioning
- Concurrent learning
- Habituation
- Self-efficacy

These are described in more detail in Chapter 10. It is sufficient to note at this point that the brain is an extremely adaptable organ, and has developed a multitude of strategies for taking advantage of information, and using it to modify itself, toward a designated end. Neurofeedback simply provides access to information that would otherwise be inaccessible, and the brain integrates this feedback into its overall strategies in multiple ways.

Classical Conditioning

The process by which an organism learns to pair two events that were previously unpaired. The most notable example is that of "Pavlov's dogs," who learned to salivate in response to a bell, if the bell had been "paired" with food. This type of learning is automatic, and does not require any voluntary behavior from the organism.

Non-Volitional Techniques

In addition to relying on operant conditioning and other learning mechanisms to produce results, it is possible to use adjunctive techniques that can accelerate or otherwise enhance the effects of neurofeedback. These may be likened to "training wheels," or coaching methods, that help the brain to find and maintain desired states without relying entirely on the ability of the brain to find and maintain these states on its own volition.

Auditory or visual stimulation (AVS) techniques are also analogous to highly information-packed coaching sessions, in which a person can, for example, significantly improve his or her ability in golf, music, or other athletic or artistic endeavor by using a "master" who can pinpoint and alter key aspects of performance. This can potentially produce significant change in a short number of sessions, as has been observed in a variety of non-volitional training situations (Collura and Siever, 2009).

Cranio-Electric Stimulation (CES)

CES is a technology in which small, but often noticeable, electrical currents are introduced into the head, with the purpose of stimulating the neural tissue, with an effect that can be palliative or analgesic in a variety of cases. CES is a general intervention, and while it may produce changes that are lasting, it is not strictly a learning technique. It is basically a way of "making the brain change" rather than "teaching the brain to change." This does not detract from its effectiveness, however, and it is efficacious and approved as an intervention for a range of mental and brain-related disorders.

Photic Stimulation

Photic stimulation consists of the use of (usually repetitive) visual stimulation in the form of LED lights or similar devices. In the simplest case, stimulation is provided by a device with a preprogrammed stimulation rate, under a program designed to achieve some desired effect. It can be demonstrated that the EEG has a response to a flash of light, called a *visual evoked potential*. This consists of a brief, transient response of the brain, in particular the primary and secondary visual areas. When the stimulation is withdrawn, these evoked responses disappear and do not persist in the absence of the stimulation. Nonetheless, there are indications that some lasting effects may be produced in the brain as a result of experiencing the repetitive stimulation.

The exact type of stimulation is known to be important. Some devices will use brief flashes of light, thus turning on and off in an intermittent fashion. Other devices use sinusoidal stimulation, and this has been demonstrated to have a more profound effect on endogenous rhythms.

Stimulation may also be locked to the EEG in some way, such as flashing on the peak of an alpha wave, or on the zero crossing of the EEG signal. Because these stimulation patterns are contingent on the EEG, they may be expected to have a greater effect on the brain than simpler, "open-loop" methods.

Results of Neurofeedback

Neurofeedback is a Learning Process

Neurofeedback is a comprehensive approach to brain adaptation and self-regulation. The brain itself creates the strategy for the implementation of the training goals. Because this method does not purport to invade or alter any particular anatomy or physiology directly, it allows the adaptive mechanisms to be natural and learned rather than imposed.

As a learning tool, neurofeedback gives the brain the unique opportunity to pair internal brain states with reward events, providing the opportunity for internal change. Because the brain has its entire repertoire of response mechanisms available for this change, there is theoretically no limit to what neurofeedback can achieve. In other words, the effects of neurofeedback are not limited to particular anatomical, biochemical, synaptic, or other mechanisms, as is the case with interventions such as medication or surgery. This gives neurofeedback the power to alter brain functioning at any level, provided only that the brain has the ability to explore the functional range of some property, and to modulate its activity in response to the learning paradigm.

As a side note, we can observe that the brain and nervous system have refined themselves to an extraordinary extent through natural processes. The minimum visually detectable signal in the human retina is equivalent to a candle seen from 12 miles, and produces a response in the optic nerve, to an input stimulation of only 1 photon per second. Similarly, the minimum threshold for hearing corresponds with a deflection of the basilar membrane in the ear, of 1 angstrom, the diameter of a hydrogen atom. These facts illustrate that the brain operates at an atomic, even quantum, level, and is not limited in its ability to process and respond to extremely small signals, by manipulating events at the level of a single atom or quantum of energy.

Neurofeedback can Implement Specific Physiological Changes

Studies of the physiology of learning have shown that there are complex internal brain mechanisms that operate at the network and at the cellular level to allow the brain to learn from the environment and implement behaviors and changes in state. These mechanisms involve interactions of cortical and subcortical networks, and allow the brain to correlate both expected and unexpected external events with internal information. This process leads to the ability to make judgments and decisions based upon the relationship between internal brain states and sensory information, and adapt the organism to the environment. In its most fundamental sense, neurofeedback puts the brain's internal state into the environment (via visual, auditory, tactile, or other feedback) so that the brain can learn to change.

Based upon our current observations and theory in the areas of human learning and physiological mechanisms, it is reasonable to put forth a position that neurofeedback is capable of enabling the brain to engineer changes at the most minute level, and make any necessary modifications to its function, and even structure, in response to neurofeedback training. Thus, neurofeedback has the potential to produce brain changes that are detailed and specific, potentially exceeding in functional and anatomical specificity what is achievable even with laser-guided surgery or other invasive methods.

The changes that neurofeedback produces are not limited to the locations specifically monitored. For example, in the process of allowing an alpha rhythm to increase in amplitude, the brain may implement changes that involve dynamic networks of cortical, subcortical, and intermediate areas. As long as the brain modifications lead to an increase in alpha amplitude, they will be reinforced. Therefore, it is not uncommon to see changes that reflect global or networked brain functional changes in response to neurofeedback training, even if the specific areas monitored and used for feedback are localized.

Neurofeedback is an Art as Well as a Science

Because neurofeedback is rooted in deeply seated issues of learning and brain modification, many qualities come into play, including expectations, sense of accomplishment, cognitive processes in the trainee, and client interaction skills of the trainer. For these reasons, neurofeedback is not a process that can be practiced in an offhand manner, in which the intervention is expected to fix the client, who can then be sent home. Rather, neurofeedback is a process in which the brain modification may interact with underlying beliefs and habits, reaction to normalization, and reactions to the subjective and behavioral changes. Neurofeedback practitioners need to be fully qualified in the handling of the disorders that they address, and must be prepared to interact with the trainee both before and after therapy to assess and work with the changes that are brought forth. This introduces an element of art to neurofeedback, which sets it in the context of other interventions, including psychotherapy, behavior therapy, and other methods in which the skills, education, and qualities of the practitioner are paramount in ensuring uniform and positive results.

Can Neurofeedback Cause Harm?

Once one accepts the basic tenets of neurofeedback, the question can arise whether neurofeedback can cause harm. Such iatrogenic effects, or "abreactions," may be observed in certain circumstances, but they must be put in context. Given that neurofeedback is a passive learning process, there is a limit to the malevolence that it can manifest. Its possible negative effects cannot even approach the toxic and psychogenic effects of many medications. In fact, one observation may be that, as the brain learns self-regulation and normalizes, side effects of medications may become evident. This may appear to be an abreaction to the neurofeedback, but it is actually exposing the negative effects of the drugs. It is a basic truth that psychoactive medications are, by design, intended for use on an abnormal brain. If a medication is administered to an otherwise normal person, it reasons out that what will emerge are mostly the side effects. Thus, if a client whose medication can cause anxiety as a side effect continues on the medication even as neurofeedback helps his or her brain normalize, then he or she may become anxious. However, the neurofeedback has not caused the anxiety—it has exposed the negative effects of the medication.

A second way that neurofeedback can produce an apparent negative reaction is if it normalizes a coping or compensating mechanism that has held the client together in the face of other stresses or other dysregulations. Thus, a chronically anxious client may show excess alpha, which reflects a coping mechanism to reduce the anxiety. Reducing the alpha will remove this coping mechanism, again, reflecting in the client being more anxious. The good thing about neurofeedback in this context is that, once the clinician understands these types of mechanisms, the effects of neuro-feedback can be anticipated and accommodated. Neurofeedback is not a panacea, a one-size-fits-all approach to make everyone feel better. It is a systematic and scientific way to introduce brain self-regulation as an essential component of clinical practice.

During my workshop, I often ask the question, "Who thinks that the purpose of neurofeedback is to make people feel better?" Generally, I get few hands on this question. The reality is that neurofeedback provides an avenue for self-control and stabilization of brain function, but feeling better is not the primary goal. Indeed, the individual may experience discomfort or other "adverse" feelings as they undergo therapeutic change. The overall goal is to restore regulatory capability to an otherwise dysregulated brain, and allow the client to find a path that does not rely on maladaptive patterns in order to cope.

It is interesting that brain plasticity has become a new byword in clinical psychology, and seems to have been recently discovered. For those who have been involved in neurofeedback since its inception in the 1970s, this is not new news. Neurofeedback not only recognizes brain plasticity as a key element in neuroscience, but it applies it directly in a manner that can be beneficial to the client.

As a final note, it should be recognized that neurofeedback, being a learning technique, intrinsically has lasting effects. It is not an intervention that claims to have immediate and singular results, and to cure all ills. Rather, it instills in the brain the ability to become aware of key processes, and to get them under self-control. Once learned, such skills can be retained, much in the way that riding a bicycle is a skill that, once learned, is not forgotten. Bicycle riding is also an apt analogy in that it integrates a wide array of sensory, perceptual, and motor activities into what the brain interprets as a single activity. In much the same way, the brain can learn skills as complex or as simple as necessary to achieve the task, and has the potential to retain that learning.

We summarize the process of neurofeedback as follows:

- Brain activity is recorded using conventional EEG equipment.
- Real-time information is provided to the brain, relating to brain activity.
- The brain exercises its potential to implement changes that produce the desired feedback. This is the process of self-regulation.
- Changes can occur in processes including cortical excitability, generation and uptake of neurotransmitters, and cortical and subcortical connectivity.
- The above changes may be specific and localized anatomically and functionally.
- Physiological changes may be validated by monitoring and analyzing EEG activity.
- Trainees may become able to retain or recover learned states without equipment.
- Trainees may be (beneficially) changed physiologically, mentally, and behaviorally.

In understanding this overall picture, it is important to understand precisely what is being trained. It is the brain that is learning, and it is learning to alter its behavior based upon EEG signals. Neurofeedback does not directly affect the trainee's mind, and it is not the "trainee" who is learning, it is the trainee's brain. In this context, the brain is basically a rather stupid organ.

It is this introduction of additional context-to-brain function that gives neurofeedback its power. Without neurofeedback, brains go about their business meeting their goals as they see fit, and this may or may not line up with the best interests of the individual. It is an important philosophical and practical point that the brain's goals are not the individual's goals. While brain goals may complement individual goals, particularly with regard to homeostasis, self-regulation, and avoidance of danger, the brain may also have goals that are counter to the individual's best interests. We may see examples of this in such aberrations as antisocial or violent behavior, thrill-seeking, or other obsessive thoughts or compulsive behaviors that satisfy some internal need but do not lead to long-term satisfaction.

Thom Hartmann (1995) has placed ADD in an evolutionary perspective by elevating the concept of a thalamic setpoint that determines the amount of stimulation that an individual requires in order to feel alive. In Hartmann's analysis, there is a final level of self-actualization at the top of Maslow's hierarchy that involves the person's need to feel fully alive. Those with a lower thalamic setpoint can be satisfied with less stimulation, and can follow a more routine or mundane life path. However, those with higher thalamic setpoints must seek additional stimulation and excitement in order to achieve their sense of being present. This is one example of a mechanism in which the brain has determined its priorities and requirements, and the person becomes the agent responsible for achieving these goals. Therefore, a thrill-seeker is obtaining stimulation and excitement based on the needs of his or her brain, and he or she is subservient to his or her brain, not the other way around. Neural feedback seeks to normalize brain function so that the individual can have the freedom and flexibility to achieve his or her goals, without the hindrances or complexities introduced by brain dysregulation.

A cat, a pigeon, and even a flatworm can respond to operant conditioning. The brain is no different. The precise mechanisms at work during neurofeedback training may not be entirely clear, but there is no need for mystery or concern that they are real. Objective results demonstrate that the brain can respond to information and alter its behavior to suit an operant goal. This does not depend so much on voluntary effort or understanding on the part of the client as it does on the brain's automatic mechanisms for adaptation and change. The brain seeks novelty and fulfillment, and will do so with or without the participation of the individual.

It is useful to speculate how many disorders may at their core be due to local optimization or goal-seeking, which costs the individual in the larger context. Among local goals is the need to be right, the need to get attention, the need to seek novelty, the need to be amused, or the need to be left alone. Neurofeedback superimposes on whatever goals the client's brain has established, the goals related to self-regulation and homeostasis, relative to healthy brain rhythms, and brain connectivity.

As an example of this superposition of goals, I recall my experience during an intensive week-long neurofeedback training with Dr. James V. Hardt. During one episode in which I was enquiring about knowing one's true motives, he responded with "ask in alpha." His point was that the brain is not likely, or even capable, of lying to itself when it is in an alpha state. Therefore, during those times when alpha was being produced in the training chamber, the brain/mind would be clear of deception and reveal what it at least thought would be valid ideas. This example illustrates the concept that superimposing an EEG condition on an otherwise normal (or abnormal) mental process adds external conditions (biofeedback) that can affect the quality or value of that experience.

This is potentially much more specific than any medication. Many conceptual and practical barriers can be overcome by taking this basic perspective. The brain is an organ, one of whose jobs (and strengths) is to modify its behavior based upon arbitrary goals. In the complexity of daily life, social and environmental pressures, and adverse life experiences, one's brain takes on habits and tendencies that can become manifest as clinical "disorders." By addressing ways in which the brain is stuck, and operating at a non-optimal manner, neurofeedback can help an individual to learn important self-regulation skills and achieve a more normalized way of functioning.

Rather than focusing on disorders and prescribed interventions, neurofeedback focuses on underlying dynamics, and how to change them for the better. In our investigation of the science and technology underlying neurofeedback, it will become clear that there is little limit on what a brain can and will do in order to satisfy a goal. When a goal is presented in the form of creating a particular pattern or amount of brain activity at a particular location, the brain will react to the goal, generally by seeking to satisfy it. This occurs without extreme overt effort on the part of the trainee.

Neurofeedback: The Big Picture

- Signals from brain are revealed to trainee.
- Brain processes new information and learns.
- Allows conditioning and change to occur.
- System must be comprehensible, intuitive, relatively simple.
- Element of volition, engagement—but not "trying."
- EEG changes may occur, but what really matters are clinical outcomes.

Clinical Uses of Neurofeedback

It is beyond the scope of this book to present a full account of the clinical uses of neurofeedback. However, some of the most prominent successes are worth noting. It should be recognized initially, however, that neurofeedback can be regarded as "diagnosis-free" in the sense that it does not have to be applied with regard to a specific disorder. Neurofeedback operates below this level of classification. It even works below the level of "symptoms," which are clusters of behaviors or self-report that themselves assume interpretation and categorization. Neurofeedback operates at the level of "function," and interacts with the brain at that level. To the extent that any disorder or complaint has functional underpinnings, neurofeedback can address that function and provide a means for change.

One of the earliest clinical uses of neurofeedback was with clients with seizures, as this work grew out of Sterman's original work with cats (Sterman, 1996). Controlled studies have demonstrated the specific value of SMR training, beta training, theta downtraining, and related protocols in this population (Rossiter and La Vaque, 1995; Rossiter, 2004, 2005).

Lubar (2003) reviewed the history of neurofeedback for ADD and ADHD, and summarized research results. He concluded that it is an established method, and that standard approaches have been shown efficacious and safe for clinical use. He also described the use of a quantitative EEG factor, the theta/beta ratio, which has diagnostic value in determining the particular type of the disorder. Monastra published a review and white paper on the use of EEG biofeedback in clients with ADHD, and provided the rationale and empirical foundation for this approach (Monastra, 2005; Monastra et al., 2005). He concluded that EEG biofeedback is an effective and important possible addition for practitioners helping children with this disorder. Thompson and Thompson (2008a) assessed the value of neurofeedback for children with ADHD. They reported on the use of the theta/beta ratios and other EEG abnormalities to help to diagnose the type of ADD/ADHD. They also reported on effective interventions using neurofeedback protocols.

Arns et al. (2009) conducted and reported on a meta-analysis of published research on EEG biofeedback used for attention and impulsivity problems. They reported a strong net effect size, and no reported abreactions, to EEG biofeedback used with children from this patient population. It was concluded that this meta-analysis confirmed that this approach was effective and safe. The protocols used were of the conventional type, being reduction of excess theta and excess high beta, as well as enhancement of sensorimotor activity (SMR). The EEG biofeedback was reported to have particular value in reducing impulsivity specifically, when this was present. This report also showed the ability to assess and diagnose the type of ADD/ADHD based upon EEG measurements.

Walker (2011) published results demonstrating significant clinical benefit to patients suffering from recurrent migraine headaches who opted to stop medication and take a neurofeedback treatment series. Ninety-eight percent of the neurofeedback subjects reported a reduction in headache frequency, while only 28 percent of the medication group reported at least some reduction. This stands as an important contribution to the field of QEEG-guided neurofeedback by showing a marked reduction in headache symptoms in comparison to medication. We would like to clarify two points regarding this study and its clinical applicability.

First, this was not a randomized, placebo-controlled, double-blind controlled study. Neurofeedback subjects were self-selected, knew they were receiving treatments and stopped taking medication. Control group members were not given sham feedback; they simply continued medication treatment. Some may argue that the lack of blindness and placebo control, combined with the self-selection process, compromised the applicability of this study by introducing uncontrolled variables (placebo, motivation, predispositions, etc.). Some might even argue that these factors compromised the strength of the result. We would like to point out that statistics show that this is not the case. In fact, this is neither a small effect nor is its clinical applicability limited to the experimental design. This study demonstrates a strong effect, which has significant clinical relevance.

The experimental conditions are valid due to the internal consistency of the design. In other words, no one would argue that what was reported did not happen. The design aspects do, however, limit the external validity insofar as the results are to be applied to the clinic. Someone might argue that the results might not apply to a headache patient chosen at random, or one who does not know which treatment he or she is receiving. Nonetheless, the study does support the following statement: "A controlled study has shown that in clients with recurrent migraine headaches who were on medication and taken off medication and opted for neurofeedback therapy, 78 percent experienced some reduction in symptoms and 54 percent experienced complete remission for over a year." In making this statement, the study has strong clinical applicability, despite the absence of blindness, randomization, or a placebo control. We also note that, while 2 percent of the experimental group experienced little or no change, no patients were reported to have gotten worse. This shows that there are minimal to no risks associated with opting for neurofeedback and discontinuing medication.

Second, we also point out the statistical significance of the findings themselves. The results were shown, but not reported in a statistical way in the report. If the distribution of symptom change shown in the report is taken as a pair of distributions, it is possible to estimate the significance of the difference in the form of parametric or nonparametric tests. From a parametric point of view, if we look at these as two normal distributions, we observe that within the overlapping tail area corresponding to less than 50 percent change, we have 28 percent of the subjects, being 24 percent of the neurofeedback group and 4 percent of the control group. If we assume a normal distribution, this amount of overlap would imply a t value in the vicinity of 4.5, corresponding to a p value of < 0.00001. Alternatively, using the chi-square statistic (40.29, 2×2 contingency, 1 degree of freedom), we again have $p < 0.00001$. One might object to this estimate, because the variables are not shown to be normally distributed along a uniform scale. If we reduce the analysis to a more conservative nonparametric form that does not assume any particular statistical distribution or scale, a more conservative estimate can be obtained. Using the Wilcoxin rank-sum test and the Mann-Whitney U test, the resulting z value is 4.25 ($U = 222$, $m = 575$, $\sigma = 83$, $N1 = 46$, $N2 = 25$), corresponding to a p value of 0.000032, which is slightly higher than the parametric estimates. This is the probability that the observed differences were due to chance. In other words, the likelihood that the results were due to random events is less than 1 in 30,000 without making any assumptions, and less than 1 in 100,000 if we assume a normal distribution. We are thus compelled to reject the null hypothesis that the results are due to chance, and conclude that the experimental treatment modality had a significant and strong effect.

Therefore, as estimated through either parametric or nonparametric methods, the reported results are significant and well beyond chance level. Thus, we are not looking at a "weak" effect; we are looking at a "strong" effect. In summary, this study shows a strong treatment effect, which has significant clinical validity and applicability. If these results are generalized, it would be reasonable to put any and all recurrent migraine patients on neurofeedback immediately, following the methods of this study. In view of these findings, the ethical considerations become significant. We can ask if is it ethical to deny or neglect to offer, or even encourage, a QEEG-guided neurofeedback option to recurrent migraine sufferers who are currently on medication. We believe that these findings show that it is not. Were these findings to be replicated in one or two additional studies, it is likely that HMOs and insurance companies could be compelled to reimburse for this treatment modality on this population, as indicated by the QEEG. Furthermore, the FDA might be motivated to approve neurofeedback for this indication, when used in this manner. We also note that the manual QEEG-guided approach shown here is entirely consistent with emerging methods that can provide equivalent operant training in a more comprehensive and automated manner (Collura et al., 2009).

Breteler et al. (2010) described the use of quantitative EEG (QEEG) to diagnose children with dyslexia, for assessment, and the use of neurofeedback to remediate brain dysregulations. This led to improvements in performance as a result of the neurofeedback training. This study used standard protocols, based upon the QEEG data, to guide protocol selection.

Trudeau et al. (2008) described the usefulness of neurofeedback for addiction and alcoholism. This included the use of different EEG characteristics to determine the type of disorder. Sokhadze et al. (2008) described using QEEG-based neurofeedback in the treatment of substance abuse disorders. The results showed effectiveness and safety.

Hammond and Baehr (2008) described the efficacy of neurofeedback in the treatment of depression. They describe the use of a frontal alpha asymmetry protocol. This provides an indication of the trend of the alpha wave amplitude between hemispheres, and allows the client to learn to change this trend toward the direction of better mood control. The amplitude asymmetry can also be used as a diagnostic indicator for depression, when used as a form of QEEG analysis.

In addition to epilepsy, ADD/ADHD, depression, and anxiety, a wide range of other disorders has been addressed with neurofeedback. Fisher (2008) described the efficacy of neurofeedback in clients who suffer from attachment disorder. Thompson and Thompson (2008b) assessed the value of neurofeedback for children with Asperger's syndrome. Ibric and Dragominescu (2008) concluded that neurofeedback is an effective intervention for clients with problems with pain. Price and Budzynski (2008) assessed neurofeedback for clients with anxiety. They reported on the use of beta amplitude to determine location and type of anxiety, and the use of neurofeedback in the treatment of anxiety.

2

NEUROPHYSIOLOGICAL ORIGINS OF EEG SIGNALS AND RHYTHMS

The EEG was first recorded by Dr. Hans Berger, a German psychiatrist. For a comprehensive summary of the technical aspects of early EEG, see Collura (1992a, 1992b)

The following recording (Figure 2.2) was published in 1932. In this initial recording, Berger was able to identify a prominent 10-cycle-per-second rhythm, which he named "alpha." This is visible when compared to the bottom trace, which is a mirror vibrating at 10 per second. He also recognized a 20-cycle-per-second rhythm, which he named "beta," visible as the smaller "wiggles" riding on top of the trace. Berger was fully aware that this signal was composed of a mixture of different frequencies, which were combined at every point in time. He went further, and pointed out that a process such as a Fourier transform could be used to estimate the frequency content quantitatively. Berger was thus both the father of EEG and the father of QEEG.

Figure 2.3 shows an assortment of possible EEG patterns that can be observed during different stages of alertness, as well as sleep. The distribution of frequencies, and the shapes of the waves, can be seen to vary, depending on what the brain is doing at that moment. While all EEG signals generally consist of a mixture of frequencies, the dominant patterns and frequency content are readily recognized by eye.

Dipole Sources and Postsynaptic Potentials

Although the EEG is recorded from the scalp, it is actually known to be produced by specialized neurons known as pyramidal cells residing in the upper layers of the cortex. The normal activity of these cells is mediated by tiny electrical potentials that are maintained across the cell membranes. These potentials are typically in the range of tens of millivolts, and can be as large as 100 millivolts or more. Each cell produces an extremely small current flow in its immediate region, but there is also current produced throughout the brain due to a phenomenon known as volume conduction.

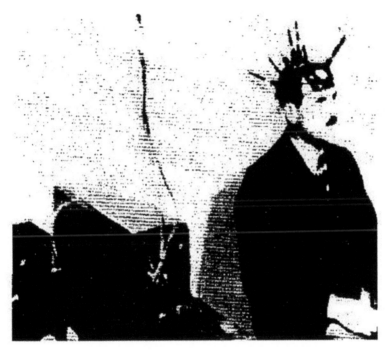

Figure 2.1 Photograph by Hans Berger of 1924 attempt at recording EEG.

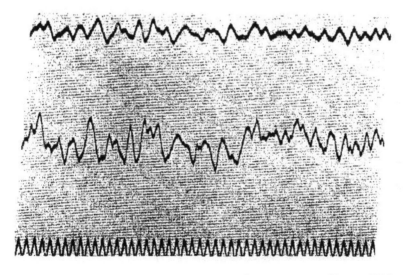

Figure 2.2 One of the earliest published recordings by Hans Berger of human EEG.

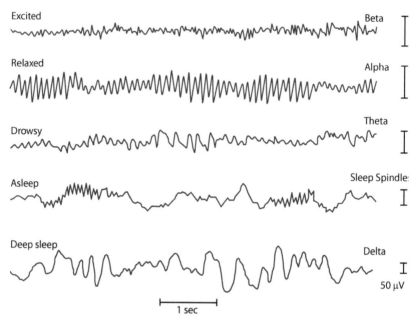

Figure 2.3 Picture with Excited, Relaxed, Drowsy, Asleep, Deep Sleep.

Poisson's Equation

The mathematical law that describes the conduction of electrical potential from the cells of the brain to the surface of the head is known as "Poisson's equation":

$$\nabla^2 \phi = \frac{-p^2}{\varepsilon}$$

This law relates the surface potential distribution to the underlying charge, and the permittivity of the mass of tissue. This provides a solution to the "forward problem," which consists of predicting the surface potential based upon the sources in the brain. When applied to realistic situations, this produces what are called "dipole fields," one of which is illustrated in Figure 2.4. It is worth noting here that multiple sources can be shown to combine "linearly," so that a combination of sources results in the arithmetic sum of the potential fields that each would produce individually.

Dipole Field Measurement

Figure 2.5 shows a realistic representation of a single cortical dipole source, in this case from the mesial temporal lobe. This figure shows the negative

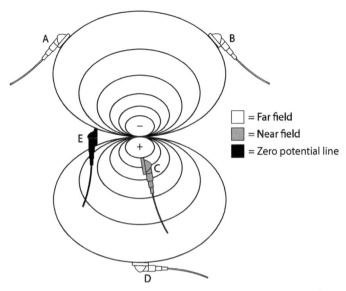

Figure 2.4 Dipole field shown with corresponding possible locations of sensors for "near field" and "far field" recording.

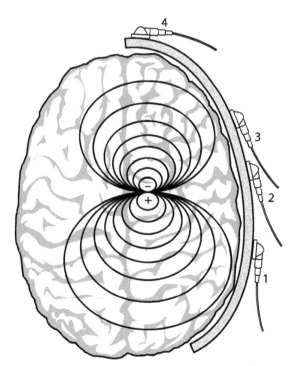

Figure 2.5 Realistic head dipole source shown in cutaway view of brain and skull, with surface sensors.

pole extending frontally (anterior), the positive pole extending occipitally (posterior), and how the field eventually reaches the scalp. Sensors placed at locations 1 and 4 would measure this dipole effectively, as would sensors at locations 1 and 3. Note, however, that a sensor at position 2 is located along the perpendicular axis, and would not see any potential due to this dipole.

The presence of a dipole such as this requires that a significant population of neurons are depolarizing in unison to produce the external potential. This is what is referred to as local synchrony. The role of local synchrony in generation of EEG rhythms is so profound that less than 5 percent of the pyramidal cells in the brain can be responsible for more than 90 percent of the EEG energy. The situation is very much like the political process, in which a small number of pivotal voters can determine an election. In much the same way that many votes simply cancel each other out, resulting in zero net result, the vast majority of pyramidal cells are operating asynchronously, so that their external potentials cancel each other out. Therefore, if only a small number of pyramidal cells begin to polarize in unison, they will be visible in the EEG. This means that the brain has tremendous leverage in altering the EEG in response to operant training.

Figure 2.6 shows an idealized view of the major cortical layers, as well as the types of cells that populate them, in schematic form. The cells are greatly enlarged, as even a small area of cortex contains thousands of cells

Cortlayers

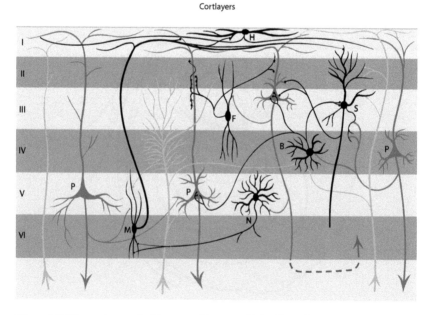

Figure 2.6 The major cortical layers, with pyramidal cells and companion neurons.

in complex arrangements. This shows the major elements of the layers, which consist of pyramidal cells marked "P" and their various interconnections to companion cells. Much of the interneuronal activity is inhibitory, exerting a controlling influence on the excitatory activity being mediated by the pyramidal cells.

Figure 2.7 shows the important relationships between the thalamus and the cortex. Thalamic projections to the cortex are widespread, and are modulated by the reticular nucleus, which exerts an inhibitory influence on these projections. Figure 2.8 further details these thalamo-cortical projections, showing how thalamic nuclei project to virtually all areas of the cortex.

Figure 2.7 shows the thalamus and the cortex together, showing how the nucleus reticularis thalami has inhibitory influences on the thalamic nuclei that project to the cortex.

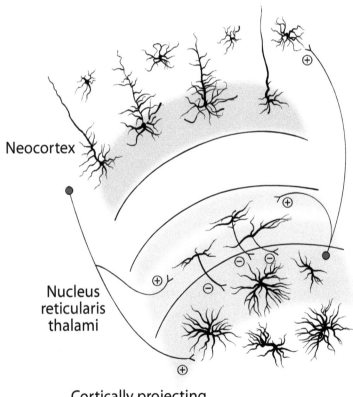

Neocortex

Nucleus
reticularis
thalami

Cortically projecting
thalamic nucleus

Figure 2.7 Thalamic projections to the cortex showing inhibitory influences of nucleus reticularis thalami.

Figure 2.8 shows the thalamic projections to the cortex. It is evident that there are widespread connections from the thalamus to virtually all portions of the cortex.

Color Plate 1 shows an anatomical view of the brain, tissue, skull, and scalp.

In summary, the EEG is generated by dipole sources located in the cortex of the brain.

Brain Dipole Properties

- Location—can "move."
- Magnitude—can oscillate and vary in size.
- Orientation—can change as sources move among sulci and gyri.

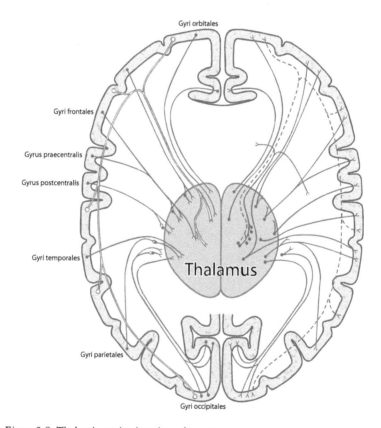

Figure 2.8 Thalamic projections into the cortex.

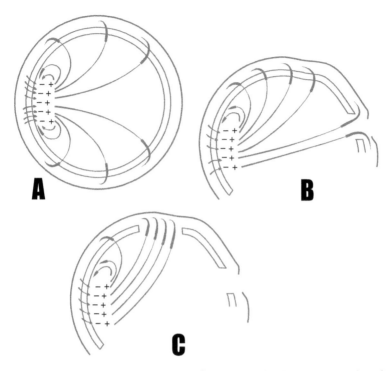

Figure 2.9 Current flow in head as a result of an occipital dipole generator, as described by Nunez (1995). In A, the current is uniform. In B, the effect of the eye openings is apparent. In C, a surgically induced opening affects current flow.

Figure 2.9 shows a realistic representation of the external fields due to an occipital alpha source, as they spread across the head. The electrical currents will preferentially flow out of any opening that does not have skull to insulate it. Therefore, the eye sockets are one location that can be used to place sensors, as counterintuitive as it might seem. Also, if there are any defects in the skull, due to surgery or injury, these areas will show abnormally high EEG. This does not reflect any abnormal activity in the brain, only the fact that the skull is absent in those locations and is not attenuating the EEG in the normal amount.

Blurring at Scalp

Evidence from Invasive Recordings

Figure 2.10 shows a set of recordings taken from the cortical surface of a human volunteer undergoing surgery (Ikeda et al., 1995a, 1995b). This was a study of "movement related potentials," and produced data reflecting the mapping of the sensorimotor system in the relevant brain regions. This provided direct measurements replicating the "homunculus" that has been so common in textbooks for decades, and shows the body distributed across the cortical surface. The sensors in this study were placed 1 cm apart, across the motor cortex. The traces shown are averaged evoked responses associated with voluntary finger movement. When the patient moved his finger, the system recorded the EEG response directly from the brain surface and averaged them to reduce the noise. This is a type of event-related potential known as a "movement-related potential." It accurately shows the brain activity associated with the movement itself. It is evident that the sensor locations are highly specific. Sensor B, for example, responded almost not at all to the finger movement. Sensor C, on the other hand, showed a large response whenever one of three fingers was moved. This shows that the brain activity is highly localized and specific when it is measured from the cortical surface.

Figure 2.11 shows the simultaneously measured scalp activity, again showing the averaged movement-related potentials. In this case, we see that the activity on the scalp surface is significantly spread, or blurred, by the volume conduction through the brain and the skull. Whereas a signal is seen maximal at Cz, for example, it is fully 90 percent of that size at C1 and C2, 80 percent at C3 and C4, 50 percent at P3 and P4, and 40 percent at O1 and O2. This shows that even localized brain activity can appear widely dispersed on the scalp. For this reason, EEG readers look for this spreading, or what is called a "field," in the recording. The field is only there because of the volume conduction and spreading, not because the brain activity is diffuse.

Figure 2.12 shows the field when drawn on the scalp surface as lines, known as "isopotential" lines (Nunez, 1995). These show the areas within which a potential that is 100 percent at Cz will appear at other locations. It is clear that a generator at that location will produce a potential that can be measured anywhere on the head, but with decreasing magnitude, as the sensor is farther away from the peak. There are several important points to be learned from this representation. The first is that any brain event is reflected at more than one site on the scalp. As a rule of thumb, 50 percent of the signal recorded from a scalp sensor arises from the brain tissue immediately below that sensor. The remaining signal is received from locations elsewhere, primarily from the adjacent sites.

Figure 2.13 shows the same scalp distribution, but assuming a reference is placed on the scalp, not at a neutral location. Because of the subtraction that occurs in the amplifier, the signals recorded referred to this reference will be smaller. The closer the sensor is to the reference, the smaller the signal will be. While this is nominally a drawback, it is still important to use and understand bipolar references in certain circumstances. However,

B

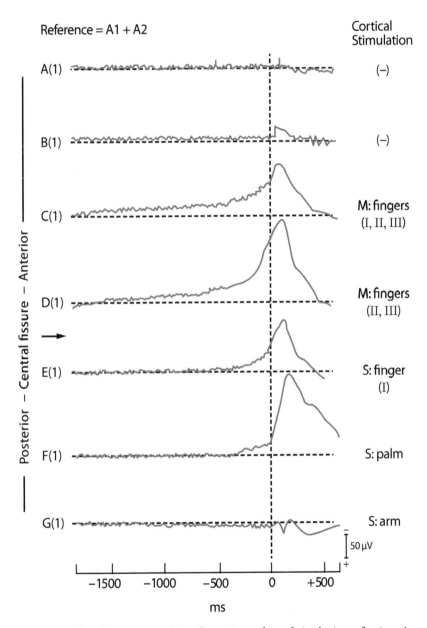

Figure 2.10 Simultaneous recordings from the surface of the brain, reflecting the movement of a finger.

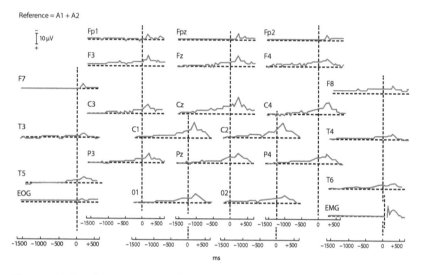

Figure 2.11 Simultaneous activity from the surface of the scalp, correlated with the recordings of Figure 2.10.

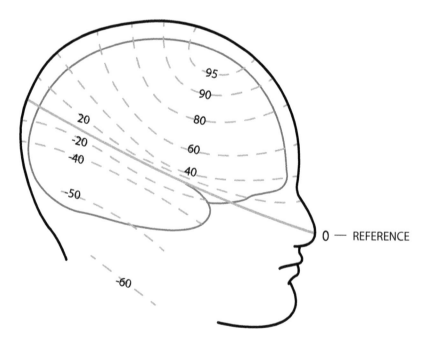

Figure 2.12 Isopotential lines due to a single generator located at the top of the head.

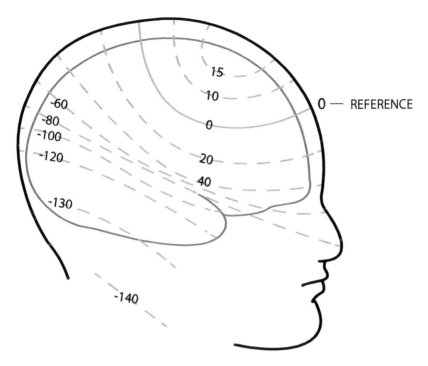

Figure 2.13 Surface potentials referenced to a reference placed on the head, producing a "bipolar" signal. The closer a sensor is to the reference isopotential, the lower the measured potential.

it is always important to realize that an active reference on the scalp will typically result in smaller signals, but signals that contain more local than global information.

Figure 2.14 shows an effect known as "paradoxical lateralization" that occurs when the EEG generator is not located directly on the outer convexity of the cortex. It is not uncommon for those beginning in EEG to assume that the dipole generators are all lined up nicely, oriented perpendicular to the scalp, as shown in part A. However, it is just as likely (more likely, actually) that the activity will be buried within a fissure, also known as a sulcus. Because the dipole is not oriented perpendicularly to the surface, a sensor placed directly above it, at w1, for example, will actually record zero potential, because it "sees" both the positive and negative poles equally. A sensor placed away from the activity, such as at w2, for example, will actually record a larger potential. EEG practitioners think about this type of thing continually, because it is critical when making decisions about surgery, for example, to know the source exactly. This is one benefit of inverse procedures such as LORETA, because they

41

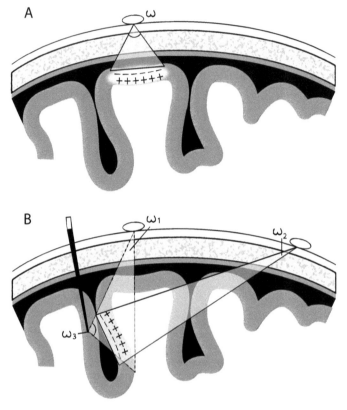

Figure 2.14 Paradoxical lateralization, in which the surface potential is offset from the actual location of the underlying generators due to the orientation within a sulcus.

"know" to locate the dipole in a reasonable location and orientation, given all the 10–20 site data.

Figure 2.15 demonstrates the surface potentials that result from a cortical surface dipole, depending on whether the dipole is oriented vertical (perpendicular to the cortical surface), horizontal (parallel to the cortical surface), or oblique (in between). There is a tendency to think of all cortical dipoles as being of the first type, so one thinks that if the sensor is located directly over the active site, then it will give the largest response. However, this is often not the case. A considerable amount of the cortical surface resides within the folds ("sulci"), and produces dipoles that are oriented differently. If a dipole has an entirely horizontal orientation, then a sensor directly above it will in fact record zero potential, because it "sees" the positive and negative poles equally. The largest amplitudes are in fact offset, and this effect leads to a phenomenon known as "paradoxical

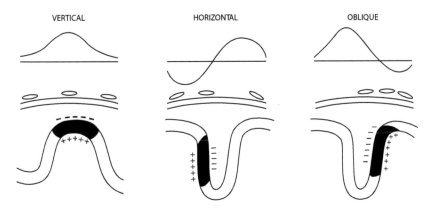

Figure 2.15 Surface potentials due to a vertical, horizontal, or oblique cortical dipole.

lateralization." In fact, in cases of the central motor strip, potentials generated on one side of the brain may in fact produce largest scalp potential on the other side entirely, owing to this phenomenon.

Another result of this effect of dipole orientation is that certain dipoles are best recorded with a bipolar montage. For example, the dorsolateral frontal lobes, active in mood and planning, are oriented so that many cells produce horizontal dipoles across the front of the skull. For this reason, Baehr et al. (2001) and others record bipolar two channels with derivations "F3-Cz" and "F4-Cz" when doing asymmetry training for depression.

Fundamentals of Neuronal Dynamics

Given a basic understanding of how assemblies of neurons can produce measurable potentials in the form of EEG, it is instructive to look at how these signals are generated from a systems and networks point of view. The brain is a complex, hyperconnected, dynamic system that relies on extensive communication and control between and among its parts. There are dynamical properties within small groups that determine how they will interact as a subunit. Neuronal subassemblies tend to operate on a collective basis, and have the ability to isolate themselves from their neighbors. This property is referred to as lateral inhibition (see, for example, Luders and Bustamante, 1990). There are also properties of how groups will interact to create the global behavior of the brain.

The cortex of the brain contains tens of billions of neurons, organized into functional groups. These groups are interconnected through a complex set of tracts that connect cortical regions with each other, as well as with underlying brain structures. In the normal course of brain function, these networks undergo rhythmic activity that occurs at frequencies ranging from one or two per second up to 100 Hz and greater. The underlying neuronal activity is occurring at speeds of thousands of hertz but the measurable external potentials are all in the EEG range.

These cortical neuronal assemblies undergo cycles of activity in which they are sequentially recruited, engaged in processing tasks, and then released. The coordinated activity of different regions is evidenced by rhythmic waves that are distinct in particular locations. This cyclic pattern of activity produces an identifiable waxing and waning of rhythms, which has a time course on the order of seconds, and also shows larger patterns of the variability. As a result, when we examine the EEG from a particular location, we can identify the dominant rhythms present, and each indicates the general state of activation or relaxation for that region.

A specific mechanism that is found throughout the cortex is that of repetitive cyclic patterns of activation involving the thalamus and the associated cortical regions. Most cortical areas are able to undergo reverberatory activity with the thalamus, which is referred to as thalamo-cortical reverberation. It is this mechanism that gives rise to the alpha rhythm, as well as what is called the low beta rhythm. By a similar but slightly different mechanism, lower frequency theta waves are produced by reverberation between the cortex and subthalamic nuclei. Faster waves, beta waves, are mediated primarily by cortical-cortical reverberations and are produced by shorter-range connections between cortical sites. All of this cyclic, repetitive activity is evident in the EEG, whose characteristic waxing and waning reveals the general state of activation and deactivation of the areas giving rise to the surface potentials that we are able to measure.

Sterman (1996) has identified key aspects of this rhythmic cycle of activation and deactivation. In particular, there is a concentration relaxation cycle, which is associated with healthy normal brain function.

The concept of inhibition is key to the understanding of brain self-regulation. If all brain connections were excitatory, there would be little opportunity for complex signal processing. For example, lateral inhibition between nearby areas is an essential mechanism to provide acuity and precision to sensory processing. Richard Silberstein of Melbourne University has emphasized the importance of inhibition by stating that it sculpts the processing details of the brain (Silberstein, 2006). In other words, it is more important where processing is being inhibited than where activity is being stimulated. It is through the control of inhibition that the brain is able to self-regulate and produce meaningful information processing.

Inhibition is a key mechanism in the thalamo-cortical regulation. The thalamus contains lateral nuclei that project from the outer regions of the thalamus into the nuclei, which then project to the cortical regions. It is these laminar nuclei (which use GABA) that provide the key regulatory function in this regard. For example, when a measurable SMR wave appears in the motor cortex, it must be accompanied by a relaxation of the inhibitory influence of the laminar thalamic nuclei. Therefore, the expression of this rhythm is also an expression of the relaxed inhibition from these locations.

What we are seeing in the modulation of brain rhythms, therefore, is the regulation and change of the inhibitory mechanisms, expressing their control on brain function. When we use neurofeedback to allow a rhythm to increase, such as when the alpha wave is trained up, the brain mechanisms at work include reducing the inhibitory influences at the thalamic level and allowing the cortical rhythm to be expressed. Therefore, neural feedback training actually has effects at levels deeper than those reflected in the EEG itself. Neural feedback is a means by which the brain determines how to satisfy the goal, and the mechanisms to do this are not limited to those brain locations that are being monitored. What is happening is that populations are being allowed to oscillate in synchrony, and the brain is modulating these oscillations in response to the neurofeedback task.

Figure 2.16 shows the concentration/relaxation cycle at the neuronal level, as described by Walter Freeman of University of California, San Francisco (Freeman, 1991). As shown in this graph, when excitatory neurons become active, they begin to stimulate their associated inhibitory cells. These cells then become active, and in turn begin to inhibit the excitatory neurons, whose activity then decreases. As the driving for the inhibitory neurons thus decreases, the inhibitory activity goes down, allowing the excitatory activity to resume again, in a cycle. This type of cyclic activation and inhibition is a key aspect of a healthy neuronal network in the brain. One key factor is that in order to maintain stable control, a dynamical system must be able to explore its functional boundaries. By continually exploring and determining its functional limits, the system can learn its stable setpoints and move between them. A system that does not explore its boundaries in this way can become stuck in one mode of operation and lack flexibility. Similarly, a system that goes into too extreme limits of behavior is also unstable. One of the benefits of using z-scores is that they "know" the normal limits for every frequency and for every brain location. Therefore, if any part of the brain is not moving within normal limits of activity, the z-scores will show this abnormal regulation.

Based upon this cycling, we can define a continuum of activity for any part of the brain. This is shown in Figure 2.17. At the left, we have the extreme case of relaxation, which is a low-frequency, high-amplitude EEG state characterized by highly synchronous, hence dependent, neuronal populations. A region that is in a theta or low alpha state is in this condition. As we move to the right, we move to the high-frequency, low-amplitude, less synchronous, more neuronally independent state. This is a beta state, associated with more "work" being done by the brain. Neither extreme is "better" than the other. A healthy brain must be able to flexibly

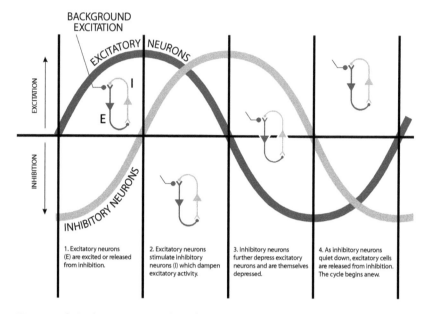

Figure 2.16 Cyclic excitation and inhibition in the cortex.

cycle between these extremes, placing different regions in the proper state of activity at appropriate times.

The importance of cyclic activation has been brought out more clearly by research by Sterman et al. (1994) on professional pilots. They were able to distinguish the best pilots from poorer pilots based upon their EEG signatures. The best pilots were characterized by shorter response times, higher accuracy, and less fatigue during a simulated visuomotor task, when compared to their peers. Upon examining EEG recordings taken during tasks, Sterman and Kaiser were able to identify a specific pattern of activation and relaxation that characterized the best pilots.

The effective pilots exhibited a particular cyclic behavior of the EEG related to the tasks. During the time in preparation of a task event, the good pilots were typically in a low-amplitude, high-frequency beta state. This was a state of readiness that suited a sufficient performance on the task. When the task was completed and the pilot received feedback, the EEG was observed to enter a high-amplitude alpha frequency state. Sterman associated this state with the consolidation of the task events, and called it the post reinforcement synchronization (PRS). It was essentially an alpha burst in which the brain was consolidating information and relaxing.

The poorer pilots did not exhibit this natural cycle. When the task event was coming, they were as likely to be in an alpha state as a beta state. If the task appeared while they were in alpha, then the pilots had to get out

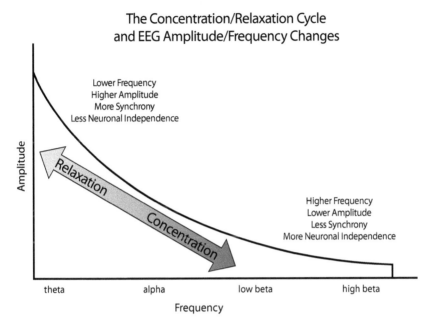

Figure 2.17 Extremes of relaxation (left side) and concentration (right side).

of alpha and enter a beta state to execute the task. The state-shifting activity caused delays in their response time, and they were less accurate because they were less prepared. Also, they were unable to exercise the PRS phase as well, which led to increased fatigue. It was thus found that the effective pilots had an innate control of a natural brain cycle that left them in maximum readiness for the task, and the ability to perform consistently repetitively.

Figure 2.18 provides a conceptual model for the EEG in a general sense. The brain can be thought of as an enormous set of neuronal assemblies, all of which are connected in various ways. Each neuronal assembly functions as a unit, but is also hyperconnected within itself, and with other parts of the brain. Each assembly has the potential to produce some measurable potential if its constituent pyramidal cells happen to be firing in unison. The scalp EEG is a cacophony, quite literally a symphony, which reflects the aggregate activity of all of these assemblies.

The brain, consisting of a network of neurons and their interconnections, exhibits control properties having to do with the production and maintenance of states, and transitions between these states. In the broadest sense, control systems either maintain states in the face of changing conditions or inputs, or facilitate changes based upon goal-seeking (Weiner, 1948). Figure 2.19 shows the basic configuration of a system-maintaining state

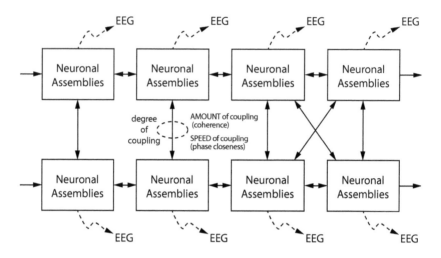

Figure 2.18 Conceptual view of the brain as consisting of neuronal assemblies and their interconnections, and the EEG as a composite signal generated by a myriad of such assemblies.

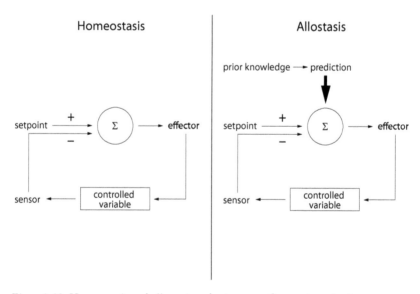

Figure 2.19 Homeostasis and allostasis as basic types of control mechanisms.

("homeostasis"), or changing output based on goal-setting ("allostasis"). It is helpful to conceptualize brain processes in these terms. Neurofeedback can be thought of as a mechanism to establish additional goals, so that the brain learns to self-regulate in new ways, thus facilitating change.

Chaos and Brain Dynamics: A Simplified View

Observations on the EEG Dynamics of Neurofeedback

There is considerable interest in the analysis and interpretation of EEG rhythms using the concepts of nonlinear dynamics, also known as chaos theory. These concepts are derived from the study of complex systems that exhibit properties such as extreme sensitivity to initial conditions, strange attractors, nonlinear limit cycles, and behavior that is difficult or impossible to predict. However, the basic foundations of chaotic behavior can be initially approached in terms of non-chaotic, linear systems, exemplified by phenomena such as simple pendulums, springs and masses, and so on. With this in mind, we can develop a model that begins with simple concepts, and provides a rationale for understanding intrinsic EEG rhythms, the ability to affect them by external or internal events, and implications for brain stimulation and peak performance training. To this simple model, we then introduce the nonlinear properties that produce chaotic behavior and identify their importance.

The Basic Model

The EEG signal may be simply conceptualized as the motion of a physical object, such as a mass attached to a spring or a pendulum at the end of a string, that is moving in response to an external force (Figure 2.19). In such systems, the key properties are the mass of the object, the qualities

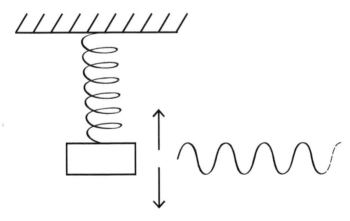

Figure 2.20 A mass connected to a spring that is attached to a rigid support will describe an oscillating motion that can be represented as a sinusoidal wave. The qualities of the wave are determined by the properties of the physical objects, and also by the nature of the disturbance that causes the motion to occur (a greater disturbance will cause a greater motion).

of the spring or string, such as length, tension, etc., and the nature of any excitation, such as an externally applied force. The salient properties of such systems are that they oscillate in a natural way in response to perturbations, they have a characteristic "resonant" frequency (or frequencies), and they require energy in order to act.

One such system is a mass attached to a spring that is perturbed by an outside force. The mass will move back and forth at a characteristic frequency, which will then die out, coming again to rest after some period of time. During such behavior, kinetic energy is manifested in the moving mass, potential energy is present when the spring is compressed or expanded, and the transformation between these two forms of energy occurs in a repetitive and bidirectional fashion. These properties characterize this model as a classical linear, second-order, oscillating system, with no chaotic behavior.

This model provides the basis for a simple analogy with a living brain. In the brain, our moving object is a neuronal mass (a recruited group of neurons) that is pooled into synchronous activity, producing a visible EEG wave. The EEG measured from the scalp is produced mainly by the coordinated activity of large numbers of pyramidal cells in (layer IV of) the cerebral cortex. (In fact, only about 50 percent of such cells are oriented so as to produce measurable scalp potential, so our EEG is an incomplete indicator.)

When a large enough number of neurons depolarize in a coordinated manner, their synchronized electrical activity produces a measurable scalp potential. The aggregation of neuronal activity in this manner can thus be considered as an analogy to "mass."

Mass, which can be subjected to motion, is produced when the neurons are pooled, and have the possibility to be fired in synchrony in response to endogenous (internal to the brain) or exogenous (external to the brain) stimulation, or "force." If a large number of neurons are pooled, this constitutes a large mass, and a smaller number of pooled neurons constitute a smaller mass. When a pooled mass of neurons polarizes or depolarizes in unison, it generates an electrical field that can be recorded from the cortex and manifested as an EEG. The pooling itself is mediated by collateral neuron networks that provide a widespread, inhibitory effect on the cells, thus modulating their firing and effectively enabling or disabling them from participating in pooled firing in response to any incoming afferent stimulation.

A Model for EEG Waves: Falling into Action

Endogenous EEG rhythms are thought of as resulting from rhythmic potential variations driven from an intrinsic "stimulus," most notably the volleys of action potentials arriving from the lower brain via the reticular activating system (RAS). The RAS in this case is serving as the agent that pushes, or pulls, the neuronal mass, initiating the cortical activity. If the RAS is inactive, rhythmic cortical activity ceases, since the cortex does not generate significant intrinsic rhythms of its own. (This is strictly true only for EEG frequencies in the range of 1–30 Hz. The cortex does have an intrinsic rhythm in the 40 Hz range, as demonstrated in decorticated tissue.) While the RAS is the dominant generator of alpha-range (8–12 Hz) rhythms, there exist several other "pacemaker" sites, including the amygdala, hippocampus, and the hypothalamus, which are involved in sleep-related delta activity and are also active in the immune system. Overall, the cortex can be thought of as containing many collections of neuronal masses that are pooled into various groups and ready for stimulation, but that generate no rhythms unless stimulated from outside the cortex.

Cortical neuron pools, like mass-and-spring assemblies, have response characteristics that include a "resonant" frequency, which is the intrinsic frequency at which they will oscillate if stimulated. When stimulated by an incoming burst of afferent activity, the cortical mass will exhibit a rhythmic discharge that will die out if stimulation is not repeated. This intrinsic resonant frequency is based on internal properties of the neuronal pool at that moment in time, and does not depend on the frequency of the stimulation. Rather, it determines the nature of the response that will occur when stimulation occurs. In addition to the dynamic transformation between kinetic and potential energy at any given moment in time, the system may contain a certain amount of kinetic, as well as potential, energy, and this will determine not only its immediate behavior, but also how it will respond to a particular perturbation.

Consider, for example, the funnel-shaped coin receptacles that are found in museums and are used to deposit donations (Figure 2.21). The coin is released at the top of the funnel, whereupon it begins to travel in a circular path around the basin, moving down the side, rotating faster and faster, in smaller and smaller circles. When it is at the top of the funnel, it takes a long time to complete each circle and is following a wide path. This is analogous to a low-frequency, high-amplitude wave such as delta, theta, or low alpha. As it moves downward, it takes a shorter time to complete each circle and is following a narrower path. This is analogous to a high-frequency, low-amplitude wave such as beta or gamma.

Figure 2.21 shows that a coin rolling down a funnel, also describes a sinusoidal motion. In this case, the resulting wave is determined by the properties of the funnel, and also by the position and velocity of the coin. At the top, it describes a large, slow wave. At the bottom, it describes a faster, though smaller, wave. In this analogy, the funnel represents a localized cortical generator, in conjunction with its thalamic counterpart. The rhythmic thalamo-cortical reverberation is conceptualized as the motion of the ball around the funnel.

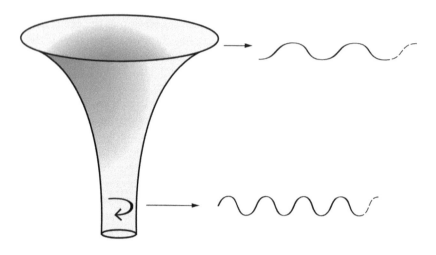

Figure 2.21 A coin in a funnel as an analogy for an oscillating system.

At the top of the funnel, the coin has maximal potential energy (due to gravity), which is released as the coin moves downward and transforms potential energy (height) into kinetic energy (speed). Traveling at the top of the funnel, the coin is analogous to a neuronal pool producing a large, low-frequency wave, and, at the bottom, the coin is producing a small-amplitude, high-frequency wave. Note that at all times the total energy is the same (neglecting friction), but that the coin's behavior, and response to a perturbation, would be different at each time. When moving rapidly in small arcs, it will be harder to change its trajectory than when it is moving slowly in large arcs. In terms of the brain, a relaxed, coherently firing neuronal pool will be more receptive to input than an agitated, busy brain preoccupied with a lot of high-frequency activity that will not let stimulation in. Note that the brain state corresponding to higher potential energy is more sensitive to differences in input, and is more able to distinguish subtle stimuli.

Once a pool of neurons has begun to act in synchrony and produce a measurable EEG signal, we say that the pool is "in motion." Like a physical object in motion, this pool of neurons can be said to have "momentum," which is proportional to the product of the mass and the velocity. It also can be said to have "kinetic energy," which is proportional to the product of the mass and the velocity squared. In order to produce this energy, one of two things must happen. Either the energy must be introduced from the outside, or the stimulus must cause the pool to convert potential energy into kinetic energy, thus springing into motion. However, a system with a lot of momentum, or kinetic energy, will be harder to change than a system that has less momentum. Moreover, a system with a lot of potential energy (such as a coin at rest at the top of the funnel) will be easy to affect, or bring into motion, with a minimal introduction of energy (simply dropping the coin).

A coin poised at the top of the funnel, ready to be released, can have a wide range of orientations. The orientation of the coin, even as it is at rest, will determine the trajectory that will ensue in response to the coin being released (Figure 2.22). If, for example, a coin is released to follow trajectory A, it will follow a circular path to the bottom, generating output A. If it is released along trajectory B, it will travel more directly down the funnel, quickly falling through the bottom and producing a less complex response. Note that the releasing action itself requires minimal energy. The orientation of the coin, combined with the shape of the funnel, is analogous to the setup of the neuronal pools by collateral neurons, which will determine the exact pools of neurons, and their intrinsic frequencies, when motion ensues. It is important to note that the starting energy level for both A and B are the same in the beginning, and it is the configuration of their basins, and the orientation of the coin, that determine the outcome, not the amount of energy imparted onto the coin. This underlies the fact that there is an effortlessness about preparing for peak performance, that the key is in organizing, planning, and releasing correcting action rather than simply increasing the level of effort or energy expended.

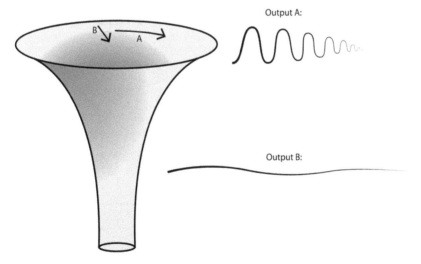

Figure 2.22 Depending on how the coin is released, the resulting wave will be different. If it is released at a sharp angle, and with a great deal of energy, it will describe an output with high amplitude, and a lasting response. If it is released directly into the center, or if it is simply dropped, it will describe a low-energy, low-frequency path as it simply falls through to the bottom.

Physiological Model and Application to Neuronal Action

Thus, preparation for neuronal action can be thought of as an orientation, in preparation for release, which requires little energy for the transformation of potential into kinetic energy, producing an automatic yet directed action. It is in the nature of a complex, nonlinear system, to be exquisitely sensitive to the initial conditions (orientation), such that the simple act of releasing can lead to any of an infinite number of possible outcomes, with a wide range of observable behaviors. Moreover, the opportunity arises for an extremely skillful and differentiated, efficient response, with a minimum amount of energy expenditure. At an extreme, a complex system can have a wide range of possible basins, separated by bifurcation points, which are stable yet optimally poised for action (Figure 2.23). These points are stable yet provide an infinite opportunity for refinement of position, orientation, and the moment of release. At such times, the brain is not necessarily in action yet it contains within it the potential for highly specific and refined action when such action occurs. Setting up the brain for optimal performance thus consists of exploring and maintaining the most efficient synaptic relationships mediating the setup of neuronal pools.

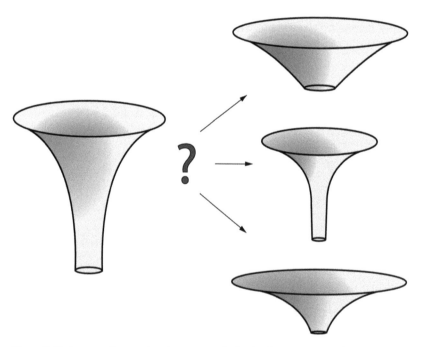

Figure 2.23 In a nonlinear, chaotic system, the basin that represents the system can change at any time, and can take on many possible forms. This variability is at the heart of the ability of the chaotic system to change and adapt its response characteristics.

What does this mean to a runner, a swimmer, a diver, a golfer, a skier, or anyone interested in optimal performance? It means that one key, being "in the zone," is to set up the initial conditions that correspond to the position and orientation of coins ready to roll down a set of basins, which are themselves determined by the current state of the brain system. When in an optimal state of being poised for action, only a minimal amount of inertia must be overcome for the system to fall into action. Thus, when an optimally tuned action is carried out, the system is really moving spontaneously from a state of high potential energy into one in which that energy is manifested in thought and action in a spontaneous fashion.

The brain builds on a repertoire of experiences that are stored, possibly at the synaptic level, and made available through the process of both conscious and unconscious repetition. The bifurcation points are the points of synaptic organization, and by developing control of the bifurcation points, and the orientation therein, the brain learns to prepare for optimal action. The information is maintained and stored both at a latent, synaptic (unconscious) level, and at a manifest, active (conscious) level, comprising the decision to execute the transformation of energies and the choice of pathways.

Walter Freeman has conducted studies on the cortex that demonstrate that the brain translates sensory information into perceptual meaning through state transitions that are determined by the chaotic dynamics of neuronal populations. These dynamics provide a substrate of neural plasticity, such that an organism can orient itself in preparation to respond to sensory input. This orientation takes the form of patterned activity that provides a "ground state" for the perceptual (and motor) apparatus (Skarda and Freeman, 1987; Freeman, 1994a, 1994b).

An example of a simple linear system, which does not reorient itself, might be a brain tissue preparation resting in a laboratory container under controlled conditions, such as used for studies of cell responses to induced stimulation. In such cases, very repeatable and predictable responses can be observed, because the properties of the brain tissue can be well controlled, and there are no unknown inputs to the tissue from other parts of the brain. In a real-brain situation, however, there will be uncontrolled changes in the system due to changes in brain and blood chemistry, and the effects of signals arriving from other parts of the brain. Thus, although at the lowest level, the behavior of individual neuronal pools may be understood as a relatively simple phenomenon. The activity of an intact brain is considerably complicated by the presence of additional influences and changes, over which we not only have no control, but which we cannot even measure.

The second factor determining the nature of an intrinsic brain rhythm is the driving rhythm that is arriving via the thalamus. For each afferent volley, there will be a cortical response that may be manifested in the EEG. In our analogy, the participant has a large sack of coins at the ready, to be deposited into the funnel in succession, producing sustained, complex responses. Coins arrive at the hand without effort, and the maximal use of brain energy is to orient the coins and to release them at the appropriate times.

An important issue is where these "coins" arrive from, and what determines their amount and nature. Clearly, the production and release of coins corresponds to that facet of brain activity that actually produces the "spins" of activity in the preconfigured neuronal masses. This is likely to be an aspect that is, to some extent, genetic, being neuroanatomic and neurophysiological in nature, but it may likely be a learned activity as well. Can we train brains to produce and "play" coins in an optimal way?

We are more concerned with the efficient orientation and transformation of energy than with the introduction of large amounts of energy. The thalamic volley is one of the potential sources of this energy. However, there are other sources of energy, both external and internal, and the critical action of the RAS is to orient and time the release of "coins," resulting in the transformation of energy into desired thought and energy. This results in the ability to detect, utilize, and transform energy into thoughts and actions. The organism is responsive to energy, whether internally or externally generated.

There are two important steps here. One is in the production of basins, with their accompanying bifurcation points, comprising readiness. The other is the orientation and release of coins in an optimal manner, producing maximally directed and efficient transformation of the latent energy into connected, kinetic energy manifested and directed by conscious (cortical) thought and action. This results in the refinement and focus of energy. For example, at one extreme, if the coin is aimed directly toward the center of the funnel, it will fall directly into the bottom, perhaps producing little observable or useful action as it does so.

The Importance of Neuronal Pooling: The Concensus of the Clocks

Because of the nature of the neuronal pooling mechanism and the properties of the individual neurons, the brain is generally not capable of recruiting a large mass of neurons at a high frequency. This is because to do so would require the existence of large numbers of high-speed pathways that simply do not exist. Fast rhythms, such as beta, are observed to occur in relatively localized brain areas. On the other hand, the brain is very capable of generating large-amplitude, low-frequency activity. Delta, theta, and low-frequency alpha waves are often seen to occur over large brain areas, often involving entire lobes. This is evidence that these rhythms are produced by widespread EEG synchronization that occurs over many brain locations at once.

In the application of peak performance, this model leads to a picture of a fit and agile brain, in distinction to one that is less so, in terms of the ability to pool and unpool neuronal masses in an optimal way. The neuroscientist William H. Calvin has developed a theory (Calvin, 1989) that explains the ability of the brain to develop critical timing, as well as planning and decision-making, by pooling large numbers of neurons into a single task. A maximally fit brain is able to pool large numbers of neurons into tasks such as accurate throwing by using what we call "consensus firing" to achieve extreme accuracy.

As an example of how pooled behavior can produce peak performance, Calvin uses the analogy of a large number of clocks. Suppose I can produce clocks with an accuracy to only plus or minus one minute, but that I can produce any number of such clocks. If I wish to be alarmed at precisely 6:00 a.m. and I set one such clock to wake me, I will receive an alarm at any time between 5:59 and 6:01 a.m. If, however, I set 100 of these clocks, and arrange an alarm to go off when the 50th of them has gone off, then I will be accurate, statistically, to within plus or minus $\frac{1}{100}$ of a minute, which is better than one second. If I use 1,000 or 1,000,000 clocks, I can achieve corresponding accuracy, with no upper limit on the number of clocks I can use. The device that counts the clocks' individual alarms, and provides a final decision, is a "consensus" mechanism, as is any neuronal mechanism that combines many cells' activity into a merged information pool.

Similarly, the human cerebral cortex contains millions of cells, each with its own intrinsic response speed and accuracy, which, as we know, is on the order of $\frac{1}{100}$ of a second, or ten milliseconds. However, human performance is well in excess of that that could be handled by a small number of such elements. For example, to accurately throw a rock 16 meters requires a timing accuracy of less than 0.2 milliseconds, which is more than 50 times the accuracy of a single neuron. By pooling the activity of thousands of neurons into functional pools, in a dynamical fashion in which "consensus" firing is controlled on a moment-to-moment basis, the brain turns itself into a finely tuned information processor that is tuned and refined continuously according to the rules of chaotic dynamics (Figure 2.24).

A "fit" brain is thus one that is able to quickly pool neurons into a specific task, and to unpool them when they are no longer needed. The mechanism of such pooling and unpooling is likely to involve the postsynaptic activity of "collateral" neurons that are able to modulate the response of neurons to afferent activity, thus bringing them into the pool (excitatory), or taking them out of the pool (inhibitory). The ability of the brain to perform this modulation can be enhanced by improving the efficacy of these modulating influences, perhaps by increasing synaptic area, increasing the number of synaptic vesicles, increasing the efficiency of neurotransmitter uptake and removal, or in any other way making the collaterals more effective in their pooling and unpooling action on their target neurons.

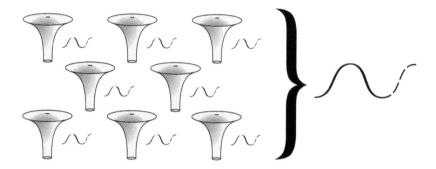

Figure 2.24 A system with many elements operating in parallel can be thought of as containing many basins. The pooled behavior of these elements provides a stability, accuracy, and speed that far exceed the abilities of any one element. A pool of synchronized oscillators produces a large aggregate signal that can be more easily detected, even from a distance.

The Transition into Chaos

The transition from this linear model to a nonlinear model that takes advantage of the concepts of chaos theory lies in the introduction of key concepts such as extreme sensitivity to initial conditions, unpredictability of responses, and changes in the nature of the response based on the current state. These would be conceptually modeled as, for example, changes in the properties of the spring, changes in the mass, or other non-ideal conditions over which we have no control, and which we may not even know exist. However, the recognition that the brain is nonlinear and chaotic does not necessarily compromise the value of these simple concepts. Rather, these simple concepts can still be applied, particularly in the interpretation of EEG trajectory data and its possible value in the application of brain stimulation, and in the development of a rationale for brain fitness training.

A chaotic system has an infinitely large family of basins that come and go in a dynamic fashion, while a linear system has a single, fixed set of basins. Thus, the possibilities in any moment of time for a linear system are fixed and predetermined, while those for a chaotic system are dynamically changing, and can be changed by learning or by the behavior of the system itself. Thus, a chaotic system can facilitate the entrance into a set of states, which are present in a latent fashion, corresponding to a state of consciousness consistent with the potential of the system (Figure 2.25).

The chaotic brain, in a state of inaction, but with the neuronal pools poised for action, can be said to have maximal potential energy. In an ideal state, the pool contains a large amount of pure potential energy, and is optimally prepared for peak performance. It is this state, characterized by high dimensionality, yet minimal action, that constitutes the rest state of

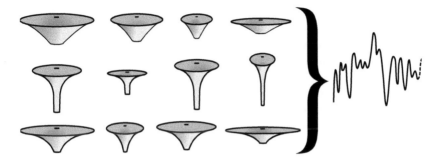

Figure 2.25 If the system is chaotic, the basins can be diverse and varied, and undergo constant change and adaptation. When the system is poised for peak action, the basins are perfectly formed, and the coins are optimally positioned and aligned. At any moment, the system can release coins, providing for accurate and efficient, yet effortless action.

being "in the zone," ready to react to either internal or external stimulation, to produce a focused, directed, well-controlled response to any subsequent input.

Towards a Clinically Useful Model

The predominant method for clinically describing brain function has historically been derived from studying pathologic brain states. This approach has been exceedingly helpful and necessary when diagnosing pathologic entities such as tumors and distinct structural abnormalities. This linear model of brain organization and function relates to many medical therapeutic procedures and treatments. However, it is inadequate for describing human behavior and more complex functions of the brain. A behaviorally specific diagnostic system does not acknowledge the reality that the whole person is infinitely more complex than the sum of behavioral and structural parts.

In their corridors and offices, clinicians acknowledge the complexity of people and their interactions. But in their attempts to communicate this to each other, many still continue to rely on a reductionistic, linear perspective. Perhaps clinicians still use this linear model because, at the present time, there is not a more acceptable coherent model available that has any meaning for relating to therapeutic approaches and treatment.

We think it is important to begin to explore other conceptual models of brain function, a model that more accurately reflects how the human being relates to his or her own physiology, as well as to the world around them—a model that helps us become healthier as we become more sensitive and responsive to our bodies and our environment.

Using a chaotic nonlinear model may provide us with greater under-standing of innovative new approaches, as well as leading edge research in EEG, consciousness, and behavior (Heffernan, 1996; Di Gangi and Birbaumer, 2000; John, 2002; Larsen, 2006). We are particularly interested in a model that can help us understand how we can optimize the potential of anyone interested in peak performance. As utilized in peak performance training, this model, derived from nonlinear chaos theory, could consist of two stages: primary and secondary synaptic training.

Applications in Training: Stage One—Primary Synaptic Training

The objective of this stage of training is to increase the potential energy of groups of neurons, preparing them to release energy in a flexible, efficient, and sensitive manner. Such properties are particularly important when these small neuronal pools are called upon to transform their potential energy into kinetic energy as members of larger neuronal pools. Primary training would typically be carried out with alpha or low-frequency training to produce a desired, controlled state of neuronal rest. But, in fact, primary training can be conducted with no frequency-specific content at all. Dan Maust (1997) has, for example, explored using wideband filters (4–32 Hz analog) in an amplitude reduction paradigm to stabilize and normalize EEG patterns in a variety of conditions.

This procedure is really not unlike the underlying assumptions of a Zen koan, in which you must let go of your attachments to a habituated way of seeing and experiencing the world in order to grasp the koan's meaning. Zen koans result in a move to a different state of consciousness and perception. All of them achieve an increase in the organism's ability to evaluate and participate in the reality of the present moment. This provides for a richer and more complex experience of life.

The high-amplitude EEG may well represent the brain's response to a traumatic or stressful circumstance stimulated internally or externally. This condition may have become habituated over time into a high "idle state" of the cortex that results in a less efficient use of energy and less sensitivity to external stimuli (although this state may have been appropriate at one point in time in response to a stimulus requiring such a high idle state). Both of these qualities described by Larsen (2006)—increased amplitude and increased variability—really represent a constriction of the ability of that nerve pool to evaluate and discriminate the stimulus, which results in a linearity or lack of sensitivity and responsiveness of the system.

The use of alpha/theta training, or of a general EEG reduction training method, reflects the goals at hand. Alpha training might be likened to a mantra in which the brain is trained into an idle, but active, state. This is characterized by a particular cycle of action and relaxation, producing the

10 Hz rhythm. To do this, brain cells are acting in a synchronous fashion. EEG reduction, on the other hand, encourages brain cells to act in an unsynchronized fashion, or to be altogether inactive. This is more like the silence in the void, rather than a mantra; it is devoid of content, but represents being poised in a pure sense, enabling a potentially infinite range of possible outcomes.

What we really want this small group of neurons to do is to be able to respond to stimuli with greater degrees of freedom appropriate to the nature and intensity of each stimuli. We would then find it to be rapidly available to participate as a member of larger pools. This model from this frame of reference (i.e. the small neuronal pools and their increasing ability to respond more effectively and efficiently to complex situations) represents an increase in their dimensionality.

The observation that an increase in linearity or the inability to have large, varied repertoires of responses to internal and external stimuli may well be directly correlated to what we perceive as pathologic states, pathology being defined as the organism's inability to effectively and efficiently participate in the complex reality of the present moment.

The result of this first stage of training would thus allow a larger number of sites to be available to participate in large neuronal pools in a more sensitive and efficient manner. It would also stabilize their rest states and make the brain more able to enter a "recovery" phase between actions. It would also have the effect of reducing uncontrolled, paroxysmal activity, including seizures.

Applications in Training: Stage Two—Secondary Synaptic Training

The second stage of peak performance training relates to the ability of neuronal pools to respond in a more flexible and non-habituated manner to more complex stimuli and tasks. Again, training can be either at a localized or at a global level. However, training is more likely to be task-specific and to be targeted at specific brain areas where secondary training is directed toward a particular goal. The same issues of increasing potential energy of the neuronal pools and increasing the efficiency of transforming this potential energy to kinetic energy are present. Various approaches to effectively train larger pools of neurons that are perhaps more specifically task-related are yet to be discovered and adopted for peak performance training.

Secondary synaptic training builds on the substrate provided by primary training. Once the brain can reach an organized state of high potential energy, the release of that energy becomes the focus of secondary training. Such training will involve higher EEG frequencies, such as SMR and beta, which are indicators of brain organization suited to application in a wide range of cognitive and behavioral tasks.

Dr. Neils Birbaumer has described and demonstrated an approach to training larger pools of neurons that he believes represents both an excitation and inhibition of attentional systems in cortical and subcortical structures (Birbaumer et al., 1990; Birbaumer, 2002). In research supported by the German Research Society, Birbaumer has shown that "slow cortical potentials indicate a state of excitation or inhibition of large cortical neuron pools." Negative slow brain potentials of several seconds in duration indicate depolarization of the underlying cortical network, and positivity reflects reduction of facilitation. Therefore, Birbaumer says "it can be concluded that self-regulation of slow cortical potentials involves excitation and inhibition of attentional systems in cortical and subcortical structures." Dr. Birbaumer has utilized biofeedback of slow cortical potentials in the treatment of epilepsy, severe motor paralysis, and aphasia.

In a peak performance model, we may be able to identify larger neuron pools, perhaps defined in "real time," while the individual is engaged in those tasks or analogous tasks defined in virtual space. Once we have defined these larger pools, we could begin to train them using models based on our EEG observations.

Secondary synaptic training will generally be organized toward the specific goals at hand. For example, a golfer might focus on occipital and premotor/motor training, while a protocol designed to enhance learning might involve frontal and occipital training in an altogether different plan. Secondary training will tend to focus on higher frequencies, including SMR and beta. One emphasis would be to facilitate the shifting from a relaxed (potential energy) state to a concentration (kinetic energy) state, with control and with fluidity. By re-entering the primary conditioned state quickly and effortlessly, after exercising a secondary synaptic activity, the brain will minimize the effects of the recovery phase and approach optimal performance.

In the design of secondary synaptic training paradigms, tasks can be broken down into neuroanatomic elements, and correlated with states of consciousness and cognitive processes. By training brain locations in specific ways, and with specific goals in mind, a protocol can lead to remediation or improvement in an identified functional area by conditioning and preparing the various brain areas and by developing the ability of these areas to interact in an efficient and purposeful manner.

Conclusions

I have attempted to provide a simple, physically intuitive model for the phenomena inherent in the dynamics of the brain during the preparation for, and execution of, finely tuned thought and behavior. This model makes use of the concepts of energy, organization, chaotic dynamics, and the aggregate behavior of many diverse neuronal pools in the production of mental and physical activity, as well as the EEG.

The breakdown into primary and secondary training has parallels in other areas. This suggests the development of individual peak mental performance according to a progression of states that starts with calming the mind (solitude, sensory deprivation), producing very low arousal states, following by stabilizing the mind (contemplation, mindfulness, reflection), all leading to a state of relaxed readiness in preparation for activating the mind (engagement, performance), which is a high-arousal state. Thus, the chaotic model of brain dynamics is consistent with, and provides an underlying model for, the emerging cyclical models of concentration and relaxation, such as reported by Dr. Barry Sterman in studies of Air Force pilots (Sterman et al., 1994).

The observed EEG signal trajectory may be thought of as a "window" into the current state of the brain, allowing us to attempt to understand its dynamics, to predict the effects of perturbations, and to develop a model of brain fitness suitable for applications in peak-performance, consciousness exploration, and the use of stimulation to alter brain states in an optimal way. A nonlinear chaotic model provides a starting point for each person to understand and experience the miracle of the complexity within each of us.

Functional Anatomy of the Brain and Cortex

Figure 2.26 shows a "wiring diagram" for the brain. Actually, this represents a mammalian brain, so these structures are common to human beings, dogs, cats, mice, and all mammals. The boxes on the top all represent cortical areas that are accessible to the EEG because they contain large amounts of pyramidal cells. When we measure EEG, we are receiving information regarding the activity of these cortical regions. The brown boxes in the middle are all thalamic nuclei, in the thalamus. These nuclei all have cortical projections, and hence communicate profusely with the cortex.

When we introduce this figure during our trainings, it is generally met with some laughter, owing to its complexity. However, it is used every day in interpreting and applying EEG data and is an extremely useful reference. By identifying the brain functions and pathways associated with different functions, it is possible to interpret EEG, as well as clinical information, in light of this diagram. A full discussion of brain function is beyond the scope of this book. The reader is referred to the excellent text by Green and Ostrander (2009) for a complete discussion of brain function related to mental health and behavioral disorders. It can be stated categorically that there is a consistent and reliable relationship between

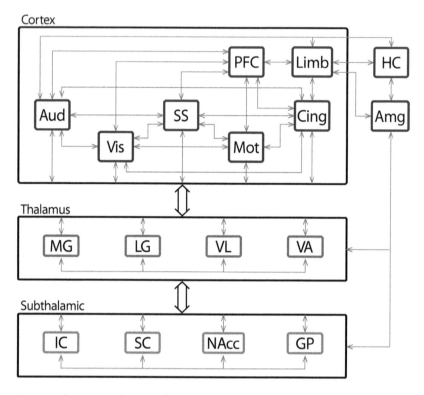

Figure 2.26 A wiring diagram of the brain, including cortex, thalamus, and subcortical and subthalamic structures.

brain locations and clinical signs, and that this relationship is essential to the responsible practice of neurofeedback. In other words, the clinician should be confident that, when specific dysregulations are seen in specific brain locations, there is merit in correlating these findings with the clinical signs, and incorporating them into the clinical plan.

Neurofeedback does not follow a simple sequence of diagnosis-specifying treatment, as is used with pharmaceuticals. It does not even necessarily follow a sequence of symptoms specifying treatment, as is becoming more "modern." Neurofeedback looks at underlying functional concerns and relates them to symptoms in a causal model. It then seeks to restore self-regulation and restore control by addressing these underlying dysregulations. Neurofeedback is not mysterious in any regard. Underlying brain functional issues that relate to symptoms, thoughts, and behaviors can be identified and addressed using an operant learning model. It is, quite simply, among the most logical, simple, and reasonable therapeutic approaches available.

For example, if a client has difficulty regulating attention and focus, and we also see excess theta in the frontal areas, then an association can be made between the two. Reducing the frontal theta would be expected to result in an improved ability to pay attention and focus, no more and no less. It will not necessarily solve all the client's problems, and it will not change the past, but it will assist the brain in self-regulating. As another example, a client who reports feeling anxious and stuck may show excess beta in the posterior cingulate gyrus. We know that this area is responsible for regulating changes in attention, and, if it is stuck in a beta stage, it is not available to the rest of the brain. Simply teaching this brain location to bring its activity back to a normal level can provide symptomatic relief, and help define a path toward more normal functioning.

The main point to be made is that the proper use of QEEG and neurofeedback requires an understanding of brain locations and functions, and how these relate to potential concerns. The bad news is that the neurofeedback practitioner really needs to understand a lot of detail about brain function, both normal and abnormal. The good news, on the other hand, is that brain functional understanding is highly relevant to QEEG and neural feedback. Studying and understanding the intricacies of brain function in this manner is an essential underpinning for the scientific use of EEG in neural feedback.

The News About Neurofeedback

- The bad news: you have to study the brain.
- The good news: you get to study the brain.

In summary, all of the boxes at the top of the figure are cortical regions, and all of these are visible to the scalp EEG. The gray regions below the cortex are the thalamic nuclei. Figure 2.8 makes it clear that the thalamus has complex and specific projections to the cortex, and that no region of the cortex is without its thalamic connections. EEG rhythms, although they arise entirely from cortical regions, necessarily also reflect thalamic activity because the cortex and thalamus are intimately connected. For example, the alpha rhythm is generated by the connection between the thalamic lateral geniculate nucleus and the occipital cortex, which is indicated by lines connecting these regions.

DC and Slow Cortical Potentials

As we look at slower and slower frequencies, there are EEG components that have been identified and are used for neurofeedback. The DC potential is the "standing" potential that includes the sensor offset and drift, skin potential, and all electrical sources. Its value is thus typically nonzero and technically does not change with time. Strictly speaking, in order for an amplifier to measure the DC potential, it must be DC coupled, which means that it is sensitive all the way down to 0.0 Hz. DC EEG amplifiers have been costly in the past and difficult to implement in digital systems. However, with the advent of 24-bit digitizers, it is now possible to acquire a DC-coupled signal and digitize it directly.

The DC potential is the actual "standing" or "zero hertz" component of the EEG. Unlike the other components, which all have a defined frequency range (e.g. 8.0–10.0 Hz for alpha), DC potentials are recorded with a low-frequency cutoff of 0.00000 Hz. That is, if the sensor is "sitting" at a steady offset of, say, 150 microvolts, then that signal can be recorded and trained. This capability allows the system to monitor the slow, graded changes in the brain potential, which has traditionally been very costly and difficult to achieve. The SCP potential is defined as the DC offset, but with a very slow adaptive baseline correction factor that eliminates the need to "zero" the amplifiers. Rockstroh et al. (1989) provide a very complete and thorough review of applications of DC and SCP signals in research and in clinical practice.

The DC signal contains all forms of offset voltage, including metal-to-electrolyte junctions, skin potential, and other offsets. In and of itself, it is of limited use because it includes so many sources of voltage, and it is very difficult to achieve stable recordings. High-quality DC sensors made of silver chloride must be used, and the physical connection must be very robust. More useful is the slow cortical potential, which is derived by removing the nearly constant standing offset, and allowing only the slow changes to be measured. In order to do this, the bandwidth of the SCP is typically taken with a "time constant" of about 10 seconds, which corresponds to a low-frequency cutoff of about 0.05 Hz, and a high-frequency cutoff of a few hertz. Most practical EEG training is done with the SCP potential. The raw DC offset is, however, particularly useful for monitoring and assessing the quality of the sensor contacts. It is thus useful for detecting poor or intermittent sensor connections, and is a useful sensor quality monitor.

The DC and SCP potentials are generated by several physiological mechanisms. One of these is the slow graded post-synaptic potentials of giant pyramidal cells in the cerebral cortex. However, these potentials typically do not extend down in frequency much below 0.5 Hz, and are primarily "oscillatory" signals. The predominant source of the slowest

66

cortical potentials is the population of glial cells that support and regulate the neurons as part of the global brain system. Glial brain cells have been found to be closely related to overall brain activation, and are also connected with brain stability. There are almost 10 times as many glial cells as neurons, and they are known to be related to general cortical arousal, intention, and are also very relevant to epilepsy and other abnormal processes. The training of slow cortical potentials has been pioneered primarily in Germany by a group at Tubingen headed by Dr. Neils Birbaumer. This group has published results with brain-controlled interfaces (BCI), as well as working with epilepsy and ADD/ADHD using biofeedback training of slow cortical potentials (Birbaumer, 2006).

DC/SCP training is generally done in a monopolar fashion. In this way, the system is monitoring the shifting of the brain potential levels relative to a standard reference. This makes it possible to specifically train the potential up or down, depending on the protocol. Unlike with regular EEG rhythms, the polarity of the training is important, as it dictates whether the brain potentials will be trained in an activating or in a deactivating fashion. This is the approach used by the Tubingen group, and is the most precise and accurate form of DC or SCP EEG. With the use of the Event Wizard, specifically directional DC and SCP protocols can be designed with one, two, or four channels. The entire DC signal, with 0.0000 Hz as the low end, can be recorded using this approach.

It is also very likely that recent use of very low frequencies in bi-hemispheric training is in fact working with slow cortical potentials. In this work, if, for example, T3 and T4 are used, the trainee is learning the effects of increasing the difference between the sensors, at low frequencies, and hence is working with basic brain activation processes. One advantage of the Atlantis system is that it permits the exact recording of the precise offset between each channel and the reference, thus providing more information than a single difference channel. It is still possible to train differences, or sums, or other derived values, based on the DC and SCP data recorded for each channel.

The DC EEG signal is rarely used in its raw form. Typically, a time constant of many seconds is typically applied to the DC-coupled EEG signal, resulting in what has been called the "slow cortical potential" (SCP). The effect of a long time constant is that, over a period of time, typically 10 or 20 seconds, the signal will return to its baseline and take a value of zero. At this point, any slow variations in the signal will be evident as deviations from this baseline. It is this slow variation in the signal that is used as the SCP in neural feedback training. Generally, the SCP is measured referenced to the ears, and is interpreted as a monopolar signal, so that positive and negative actually mean something different in terms of cortical activation. Signals that are "surface negative" are associated with activation, while signals that are "surface positive" are associated with deactivation.

It is believed that, in contrast to typical EEG signals that are generated by postsynaptic potentials in pyramidal cells, SCP signals are at least partly generated by the glial cells that abundantly populate the cortex. Glial cells are more involved with overall activation and regulation of brain function than specific information processing, so they reflect a different dimension of brain activation than the normal EEG signals (see Color Plate 2).

Therefore, it is possible to train SCP signals in a given direction, and this is the general paradigm. In fact, in SCP research and neural feedback, the trainee may be asked to cause the slow potential to go either up or down, depending on the task. It has been found that trainees can learn to voluntarily shift their SCP in the desired direction upon command,

A third category is the "infra-low frequency" (ILF) or "infra-slow fluctuation" (ISF) EEG, which is recorded by using the lowest possible reach of an AC-coupled amplifier. While it can be argued that this signal is essentially a type of SCP, the manner of measurement and recording is still different. There is some controversy surrounding whether or not this is an appropriate approach. However, the reality is that, when looking for specific shifts in slow potentials, an AC-coupled amplifier can still reflect such changes in its output, if at a significantly reduced level.

Given that there is an equivalence between the filter time constant and its lower cutoff frequency, the response of an EEG amplifier at the low end can be specified in either way. For example, a low-cutoff frequency of 0.05 Hz is equivalent to a time constant of about eight seconds. Since it takes a system about three time constants to complete a shift from one level to another, this filter would take about 24 seconds to complete a full response to a sudden shift. However, in biofeedback applications, a threshold is set that is much lower than the expected total shift, so that response is much more rapid. ILF training amounts to watching for a sudden shift in the EEG baseline and rewarding it. As a practical consideration, most ILF training is done with a bipolar channel, typically using T3 and T4 as the active and reference. Therefore, ILF training done this way rewards any change in the EEG baseline, in any direction, and does not discriminate the direction of the change. This aspect distinguishes this training from the more typical forms of DC and SCP EEG and biofeedback.

Both objectively and subjectively, DC and SCP potentials are a thing apart from conventional EEG rhythms. Color Plate 3 shows the relationship between SCP and DC signals for a typical shift occurring over a period of one minute. Color Plate 4 shows an SCP signal simultaneous with the magnitude of a theta wave. An SCP signal does not resemble the magnitude of an alpha or SMR wave, which waxes and wanes continually. When using conventional EEG magnitudes, the trainee must learn to let go and allow the feedback to lead the brain into a state that is often difficult to articulate. Some experienced peripheral biofeedback practitioners struggle when confronted with the apparent uncontrollability and relentless waxing and waning of EEG magnitudes. Slow cortical potentials, on the other hand, have a different "flavor." When using SCP signals, there appears to be more of a tendency for there to be essentially no response at all, until the brain decides to do something interesting. Monitoring four channels allows the simultaneous observation of all four brain quadrants.

When demonstrating four-channel SCP monitoring and training, trainees may report that, after a few minutes, they become aware of something to do with intention and the relationship to the environment, which shows up in SCP signal deflections. For example, when an interesting discussion begins, one or more of the traces may rise for many seconds, reflecting the change in regional brain activation. By observing the location and direction of the shift, it is possible to observe brain responses in real time that are not possible using conventional EEG rhythms. When using a standard F3/F4/P3/P4 montage, the responses may reflect regional hemispheric function, roughly corresponding to the following (see Color Plate 4):

- F3: Approach, engagement, interest.
- F4: Withdrawal, apprehension, disinterest.
- P3: Language processing, integration with self, logical reasoning and memory.
- P4: Image processing, integration with environment, spatial reasoning and memory.

Color Plate 5, for example, shows F3 and F4 SCP data over a period of five minutes. It is apparent that, at times, the entire frontal cortex is shifting in a similar fashion, demonstrating hemispheric coordination of activation patterns. At other times, however, they clearly behave separately, revealing differential hemispheric activity. Color Plate 6, similarly, shows F3 and P3, demonstrating intra-hemispheric slow cortical potentials and their relationship.

DC and SCP potentials provide a valuable window into the brain and mind, and one that has historically been difficult and costly to obtain. With new technology, it is now possible to record and train DC and SCP brain signals in any clinical or research environment.

Figure 2.27 summarizes the possible range of low- and high-frequency signals that can be extracted from the EEG, depending on filter settings. DC, infra-slow fluctuations (ISF), slow cortical potentials (SCP), and the typical EEG are all derived from the same basic signal.

Figure 2.28 is a typical whole-head from 19 channels, viewed as a six-second recording. A complete discussion of the EEG is well beyond the scope of this book, so the reader is referred to the excellent text by Neidermeyer and Lopes da Silva (2005). The basic message at this point is to understand that the EEG consists of a set of surface potential

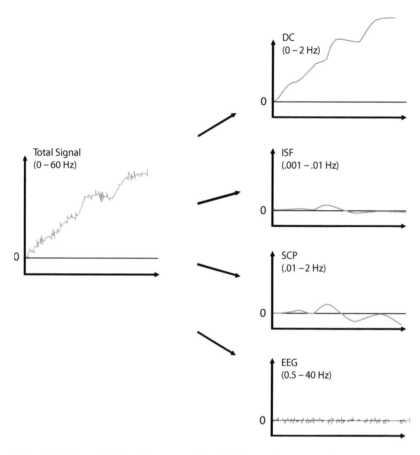

Figure 2.27 A raw EEG and a range of signals that can be measured.

measurements that reflect the underlying brain activity, mixed in with some muscle and eye artifact as well. A healthy EEG reflects the flexibility and variety of frequencies as shown here, while still having an organized appearance. Learning to read EEGs simply takes repeated exposure, and is well worth the effort.

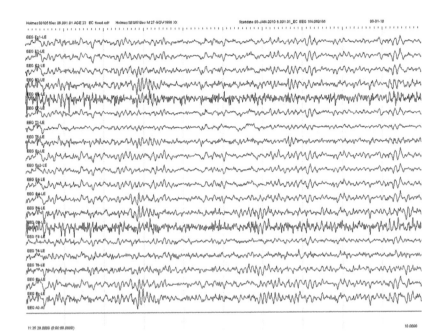

Figure 2.28 A typical EEG, showing the mixture of fast and slow frequencies and the waxing and waning of different components.

3

EEG INSTRUMENTATION
AND MEASUREMENT

Introduction

The heart of neurofeedback is the measurement of the EEG signal from the scalp. Therefore, it is important to understand the principles of EEG and how the scalp measurements reflect brain activity. As previously explained, brain electrical events produce tiny, but measurable, electrical potentials at the surface of the scalp. Although the brain potentials are on the order of 100 millivolts, by the time the signals reach the scalp the amplitudes are reduced by a factor of over 1,000. Therefore, scalp potentials are on the order of microvolts (millionths of a volt). In order to measure these tiny potentials, it is necessary to take special precautions in the design and use of very sensitive amplifiers. The fundamental property of a suitable biological amplifier (Figure 3.1) is that it is a differential amplifier. That means that it amplifies the difference between two sites and produces that difference signal as the output.

Differential Amplifiers

A differential amplifier is important because the subject's body (and head) is awash in electrical noise, both from within and without the body. Signals that comprise extraneous noise are generally the same or similar all over the body because they are spread throughout the subject's tissue. In order to measure the activity of a specific region, such as the cortex of the brain, the amplifier must be able to pick up the difference between the sites and reject the common signal. This ability to amplify the difference and reject the common signal is quantified as the "common mode rejection ratio," known as CMRR. In a practical EEG device, the CMRR must be 100 dB (decibels) or more, meaning that the differential gain must be 100,000 or more times larger than the common-mode gain. This allows the amplifier to tolerate noise many times larger than the actual signal, while still rejecting it.

When the differential amplifier is applied to the scalp, the model in Figure 3.2 can be used to understand the electrical events that produce the

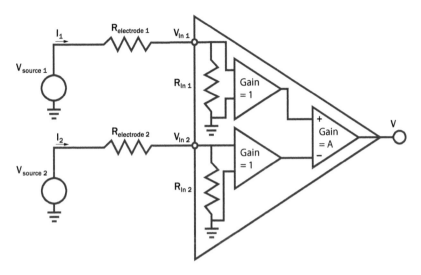

Figure 3.1 A differential amplifier of the type used in bio-potential measurement.

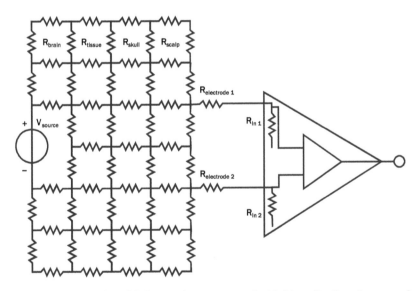

Figure 3.2 The head modeled as a voltage source embedded in a distributed system of resistances, connected to a differential amplifier.

EEG. We use the network of resistors to represent the "distributed" resistance of the brain and head. The electrical currents produced by the voltage source (at left) pass through the distributed resistances, getting smaller and smaller, until they appear at the surface of the scalp, on the right side of the array. The amplifier then picks up the scalp signals and amplifies them to produce the EEG. Therefore, the connection between brain activity and the EEG is well understood, and there is no mystery or uncertainty regarding the generation of the signal used to control neurofeedback. It is hoped that this explanation can help to separate neurofeedback from other fields in which the mechanisms are much less clear, and which may need to resort to "categorical" arguments to justify their effects. EEG is, quite simply, the most direct and objective means of measuring the electrical activity of the brain without actually going inside the head with invasive sensors (as we saw in Chapter 2).

As an example of a specific EEG measurement, consider Figure 3.3. The dipole represents a realistic source, and would, in this example, be located in the mesial right temporal lobe. It is oriented toward the front and back, in what is called an anterior-posterior orientation. As a result, an amplifier that has one sensor in the right front of the head, and another sensor in the right rear, will be able to "see" this dipole. If, for example, the (+) sensor picks up a potential of 5 microvolts, and the (−) sensor picks up a potential of −3 microvolts, then the resultant signal would be 5− (−3) = 8 microvolts.

It should be understood that, in normal circumstances, the desired EEG signal is not free of interference, but is "riding on" a combination of offset, drift, and noise. For example, the sensor interface to the skin is not passive, but has its own tiny electrical activity, which may include DC offset and drift. Also, whatever electrical noise is in the room will also be passing through the body of the client, and can interfere with the EEG recording. Therefore, EEG recording is always done in a differential fashion, in which two inputs to each amplifier are used, and the inputs are subtracted from each other.

Given the ability of the amplifier to measure the difference between two sites, it is important to keep this in mind in interpreting EEG signals. When all you have is the difference between two numbers, you lose certain information. Among the most important factor is that, when the EEG signal is small, there is more than one way to create that result. As shown in Figure 3.4, an EEG signal that is zero (or small) can result either when both inputs are small, or also whenever both inputs are the same (or close). Conceptually, this is a "many-to-one" problem, in that many possible input signals can produce a particular output. Therefore, when looking at an EEG signal, it is not generally possible to determine what the underlying activity is, unless additional channels are acquired, and it is possible to carefully analyze all the input combinations.

This is particularly significant when using "bipolar" connections, so that both the active and reference are potentially active. In the case of bipolar training, if any component is being downtrained (rewarded for being lower), then the brain can adopt one (or both) of two strategies to satisfy the feedback. One is to reduce the amplitude on both sites monitored. The

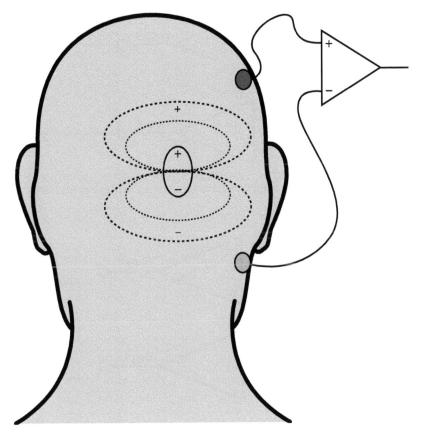

Figure 3.3 Head model containing a dipole source, connected to a differential amplifier.

other, however, is to synchronize the two sites and allow the activity to persist. This fact likely contributes to the fact that bipolar downtraining may be less predictable than monopolar training (Fehmi and Collura, 2007).

Figure 3.5 demonstrates further the fact that, when an event is visible on the output of an EEG amplifier, there are many ways to achieve a given result. In this case, a single upgoing peak is seen in the output. One way to produce this would be to have both signals be the same, and for input 1 to have an extra positive "excursion." Another would be for channel 1 to be silent, and for input 2 to have a negative "excursion." All possible intermediate signal combinations can produce this one output. Therefore, there are an infinite number of possible inputs that can produce any given output. This makes the choice of references important for neurofeedback. Often, a "linked-ears" reference will be used, as this provides a well-defined and reasonably quiet reference.

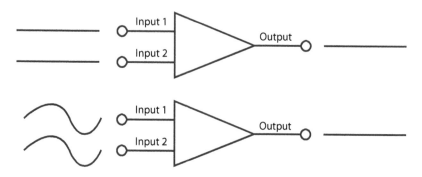

Figure 3.4 Possible inputs to a differential amplifier showing zero (or very low) output.

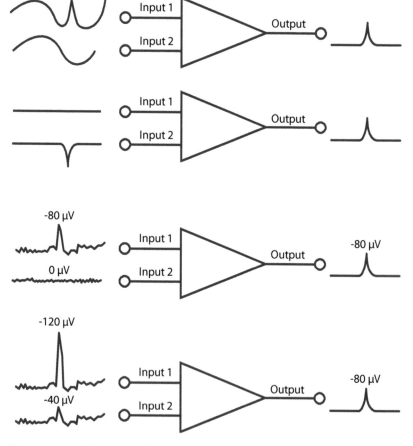

Figure 3.5 Amplifier outputs for various input configurations. It is possible to obtain a given output in many ways.

These are simple cases showing that, when we have a differential measurement, we can never be sure of the underlying signals. The real problem actually goes much deeper than this, however. These examples serve to highlight a very important general principle: the distinction between what is called the forward problem and the inverse problem. The forward problem in brain physiology states that given the sources of electrical potential and the anatomical structures, it is possible to predict the external potentials, including the surface scalp potential. The forward problem has been solved for many years, and it is known that a single solution exists for any set of sources and anatomy. This is called a deterministic solution, and this solution shows us that we understand completely how electrical potentials from neurons can produce the electrical signals we see at the surface.

The alternate problem, the inverse problem, is not so simple. Given a set of surface potentials, we want to find the sources and their anatomical locations that give rise to the signals. As it turns out, this is not only difficult, but in some ways impossible to solve. For example, for any given surface distribution, it can be shown that there are many possible source configurations that could lead to this potential distribution. This means that, given any set of EEG surface potentials, we cannot determine for sure what the underlying story is. We shall see later that a practical approach to this problem exists in the form of various inverse solutions, including LORETA. However, these solutions depend on certain assumptions that lead to a particular solution. Therefore, it should always be kept in mind that although we completely understand the mechanisms that give rise to the surface EEG, we are, in principle, only able to estimate the underlying sources and can never be 100 percent confident in any calculation that produces this type of result.

EEG Sensitivity

- Picks up difference between active and reference via subtraction.
- CMRR—common-mode rejection ratio measures quality of subtraction.
- High CMRR rejects 60 Hz, other common-mode signals, amplifies difference.
- Sensor pair picks up dipoles near sensors, between sensors, and parallel to sensor.

An important result of these considerations is that the EEG amplifier, with its two sensor positions, will pick up brain dipole sources that are between the sensors, close to either sensor, and oriented parallel to the sensor axis. These three conditions determine the regions from which signals will optimally be detected by a sensor pair.

In Figure 3.6, we are visualizing the region of maximum sensitivity for a sensor placed on the right top of the head (actually near "C4"), referenced to the right ear. As seen here, the area of maximum sensitivity actually skirts the surface of the head somewhat, and favors dipoles that are oriented "up and down," hence those that would be more parallel to the cortical surface. This is the result of what is called an "ipsilateral" ear reference.

Figure 3.7 shows what happens when a "contralateral" ear reference is used. In this case, the favored brain sites lie more deeply in the cortex and are perpendicular to the brain surface. This connection, therefore, often results in larger signals than the ipsilateral reference. While this might be counterintuitive to some, it is validated in practice, and illustrates the properties of volume conduction and dipole localization.

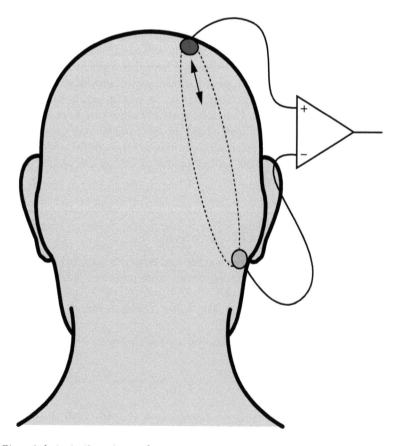

Figure 3.6 An ipsilateral ear reference.

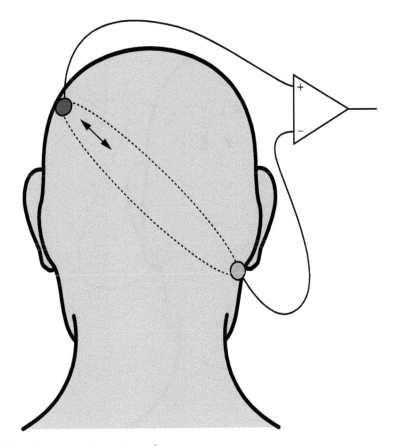

Figure 3.7 A contralateral ear reference.

Figure 3.8 shows the use of a "linked-ears" reference. In this case the two ears are connected (either electrically or in computer software) to produce a reference that reflects the entire bottom of the brain. As a result, different scalp locations tend to have a more uniform view of the brain activity. The connection of the ears has the effect of producing an equal potential ("isopotential") across the base of the brain. This is an artificial situation, and is one reason that this method has its detractors. However, it is a stable and repeatable reference that is widely used in QEEG, and has become a standard for live z-score training in particular.

In practice, EEG signals are often recorded to an arbitrary reference, such as A1, or even Cz, and reformatted in the computer. With the availability of software with this capability, the actual recording reference becomes less of an issue. However, the reference used for EEG viewing, QEEG processing, and neurofeedback remains a critical decision that needs to be carefully considered and chosen in practice.

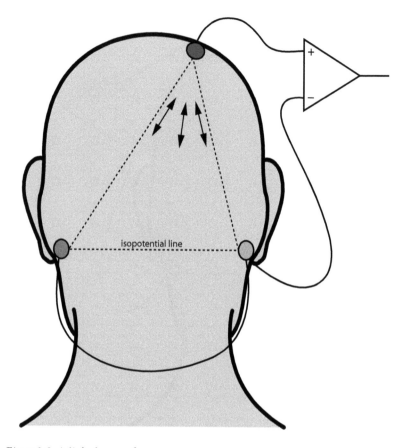

isopotential line

Figure 3.8 A linked-ears reference.

EEG Signal Characteristics

- Microvolt levels—typically 5–50 microvolts.
- Monopolar or bipolar sensor placement.
- One or two channels (or more).
- 0.5–40 Hz typical, more recently 0.0–60+.
- "Composite" wave—combines all brain activity into a single wave from each site.

The 10-20 System

This system is a standardized and accepted method for identifying locations on the scalp for EEG recording. It was developed early on by EEG pioneers, and is based on taking measurements of the head and assigning locations based upon prescribed distances along the measurements. The naming system includes the letters "F" for frontal, "C" for central, "P" for parietal, "T" for temporal, and "O" for occipital.

In this system, the odd-numbered locations are on the left side of the head, and the even-numbered positions are on the right side of the head. The name 10-20 comes from the fact that the sensor spacings are defined as 10 percent or 20 percent of the measure distance of the head. The 10-20 system includes 19 sites, consisting of eight left-sided, eight right-sided, and three central sites. The neural feedback practitioner should become very comfortable with this system as it is used on a daily basis and is essential for standardizing assessments and training, and for communicating results.

In addition to the two inputs, any practical amplifier also requires a "ground" input that allows current to flow between it and the active or

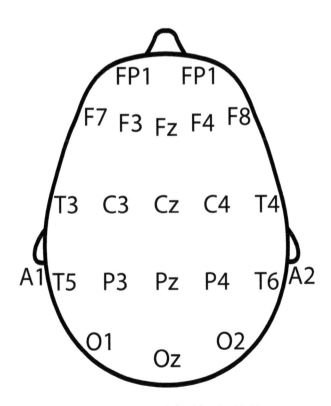

Figure 3.9 The standard sensor positions defined by the 10-20 system.

reference lead, allowing the amplifier to operate. Therefore, for single-channel work (one active, one reference, one ground), three sensors are required. When two-channel work is done, an additional active and reference are generally used, providing a total of five sensors.

Figure 3.10 shows the basic connections for one-channel and two-channel monopolar EEG. The possible variations on these are endless. However, all EEG systems require these basic elements, which consist of the placement of active sensors somewhere on the head, as well as reference and ground connections.

The top figure shows a basic one-channel "monopolar" connection. The EEG from the top of the head is being recorded with reference to the left

Basic 1-channel connection:

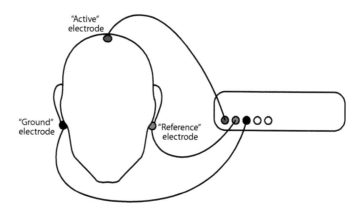

Basic 2-channel connection:

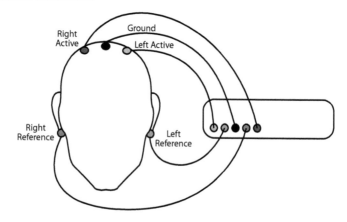

Figure 3.10 Basic one-channel and two-channel sensor connections.

ear. The right ear is used as the ground and does not enter into the measurement. The bottom figure shows a basic two-channel connection. In this example, the left active sensor is measured relative to the left ear and the right active sensor is measured relative to the right ear. This is just one of several options, but represents a common starting point for two-channel work. Another common option is to connect or "link" the ears so that they are at the same potential. While this has its own concerns, it at least provides a uniform reference. Linked ears in this situation would, for example, be used for a mini-assessment or for live z-score training.

EEG Sensor Materials

Ultimately, the measurement of the EEG amounts to sensing the potential (voltage) on the surface of the skin, and this requires an electrical connection. Also, some current flow is required in order to convey the voltage, in accordance with Ohm's law. This is the reason for the ground connection in all EEG systems. The current flow in the ground can be extremely tiny, on the order of microamperes or less, but it must be present nonetheless for the amplifiers to operate. The requirement for this electrical connection requires EEG practitioners to ensure a good physical connection to the client, with proper use of preparation of the skin area, and use of a paste or gel. (Dry EEG sensors are appearing, but these generally still require a tiny current flow across the skin boundary and also incorporate amplifiers placed directly on the sensors.)

Any sensor, regardless of the material, must be attached in some way to the scalp. This is often achieved with a paste or adhesive gel. In this case, the paste itself is also the electrolyte that conveys the EEG currents. In other cases, a cup-type sensor may be used, into which gel is injected. A cup may be attached with a physical band or cap, or glued on with gauze and collodion (this latter method is costly, noisy, and uncomfortable, but is widely used in hospitals and EEG clinics). There is a wide variety of caps, bands, headphones, and other appliances designed to attach EEG sensors. None of them are ideal, and the ones that work better tend to be more costly. Therefore, practitioners tend to find what works best for them and to stay with it.

The selection and use of sensors is one of the areas in which neurofeedback is an art as well as a science. There is no global consensus on these issues, and decisions are influenced by a variety of factors. These include budget, clinician preference and style of working, the comfort of the client, and the type of results desired. If only one or two channels are to be used, then "free" sensors at the ends of individual lead wires may be used and affixed with paste. Alternatively, a simple band may be used to hold them in place. Some bands are comprised of fabric or Velcro. Another strategy is to use a fabric wrapper or wick into which the sensor is inserted. In these cases, an electrolyte solution, or even optic solution, can be used as the electrolyte. The reality is that almost anything that contains salt, either sodium chloride or potassium chloride, will provide a suitable electrolyte for bio-potential recording.

The use of electrode caps for whole-head work or for MINI-Q applications is also very common, but not without its issues. Caps that include the 10-20 sites are relatively convenient and allow the practitioner to avoid having to measure the head. However, connections are not always guaranteed to be good, and physical issues such as "buckling" of the fabric may be a concern. Also, if one sensor breaks, then the entire cap must be repaired or discarded. Some clients, particularly children, may not tolerate an electro-cap or any type of appliance on the head. Simple cloth caps may be as little as $200, while more elaborate caps or assemblies can be $1,000 or more. A different size unit is generally needed for different head sizes, so two, three, or more caps must be on hand. They must also be cleaned and dried between clients. One reason for increased use of caps is the development of whole-head QEEG-based assessment and training, which can provide rapid results, thus justifying the use of a cap. Generally, it is the author's experience that hospitals doing conventional EEGs do not gravitate toward any type of cap or assembly, and prefer manual measurements and placement of "free" sensors, generally gold-plated.

A variety of sensor materials are used for EEG applications. Technically, the sensor material is not making contact with the skin directly. There is always an electrolyte solution that mediates the transfer of ions. While electrical current is carried by electrons in the lead wires, electrons cannot flow from the sensor material into the skin. Therefore, there is no direct contact with the skin. Instead, ions mediate the flow in and out of the electrolyte solution or paste, and this is what completes the circuit. It should also be noted that the sensor material, which is usually some form of metal, also has its own electrolytic behavior when in contact with a solution. Therefore, different materials produce their own small but important levels of noise. It is thus desirable to use a sensor material that has low noise and is also either of relatively low cost or extremely durable.

It should be noted that sensor materials should not be mixed in an EEG application. That is, only one type of sensor should be used, for active, reference, or ground leads. If one material is different from another, a variety of problems can arise. The most notable is that the difference in metals can produce an electrolytic reaction, resulting in an offset potential, and possibly drift. As a typical example, if an electrode cap uses tin sensors but the earclips used are gold-plated, then there will likely be a large DC offset superimposed on the signal. While this offset may go unnoticed in some cases, it can cause problems with DC-coupled amplifiers and can also produce a drift signal due to slow changes in the sensor polarization characteristics.

All sensor materials except for silver chloride provide a "metallic" connection, which means that there is a metal in contact with the electrolyte solution. A layer of ions invariably forms at this layer, producing a capacitive effect. When sufficient ions have built up, no further current is possible, so the sensor interface blocks DC, as well as low frequencies. Therefore, while various metal sensors are acceptable and used commonly for clinical EEG, none of them suffice for DC or low-frequency work, except for silver chloride or carbon. Carbon sensors are very rare, and act on the principle of having an enormous surface area that accommodates a large buildup of ions without blocking current flow.

Figure 3.11 shows the basic chemistry that is at work when a typical sensor material is used. The "cations" are typically sodium or potassium, and the "anion" is typically chloride. Because these ions cannot physically enter or leave the sensor material, there is a buildup of ions in the electrolyte solution. These form a layer that is effectively a capacitance, blocking the standing or DC potential. Therefore, typical sensors provide only an AC-coupled connection and cannot accurately record DC or very slow potentials on the order of 0.01 Hz or below.

Tin (Sn) sensors are among the most economical, and are often used, particularly in connection with electrode caps or harnesses. Tin is readily stamped or machined and is easily connected to the leadwire material. It has moderately good performance, and is suitable for general QEEG work. However, it is not useful for DC or SCP due to its tendency to polarize, and thus block, low-frequency currents.

Gold (Au) sensors are a preferred material in many situations. Usually, sensors are gold-plated over a base of tin or nickel (Ni). Gold has good noise performance, and is a durable material. Care must be taken to avoid abrading or wearing away the gold plating, as this would then result in a

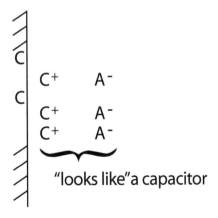

Figure 3.11 Sensor boundary with ion layer buildup.

bimetallic situation. However, rugged and reasonably affordable gold-plated sensors are available, and are standard with several manufacturers. In particular, when "free" electrode attachment is used, gold sensors are a good choice. Many hospitals continue to use individual gold sensors, affixed with collodion and gauze and filled with gel, as a clinical standard.

Silver (Ag) can also be used as a sensor material, but its use is controversial. Silver sensors may be prone to noise, particularly high-frequency noise. Historically, silver sensors have been costly and considered a premium. It has been more typical when using silver sensors to treat them with "chloriding," described below.

Figure 3.12 shows the chemistry of a sensor boundary when silver chloride (AgCl) sensors are used. Because both ions are capable of both entering and leaving the sensor material, current flow is possible in both directions, and it is also possible to pass DC current continuously across the boundary.

Silver chloride is an ideal sensor material, and is the only material other than carbon that is capable of exchanging ions continuously, thus facilitating DC or SCP recording. AgCl is also among the lowest-noise sensor materials because the exchange barrier is free of metallic reactions. It is generally accepted that AgCl is required for work with DC or SCP potentials. There are two basic approaches to producing AgCl sensors. One is to start with a silver or silver-plated disk and then cover it with silver chloride using an electrolytic process. This can be as simple as placing two sensors in a solution of salt (sodium chloride, NaCl) and applying a small electrical potential using a battery. In this case, one sensor becomes plated with a coating of silver chloride, while the other sensor gives up silver to the solution. This process can be an inconvenience, and the silver chloride can also wear off in time, requiring repeated chloriding operations.

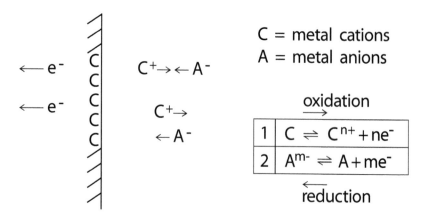

Figure 3.12 The chemistry of a sensor boundary when silver chloride sensors are used.

Laboratories that use this approach typically have a chloriding "setup" continually available for use.

A more practical but technologically more complex approach is to produce sensors of silver chloride directly. AgCl in its native form is a powder, so some physical processing is necessary when producing sensor disks. The most common method has been to press a powder consisting of a mixture of silver and silver chloride into a disk, using a process called "sintering." The mixture is required because the silver actually conducts the electricity from the leadwires, while the silver chloride is the active agent that exchanges ions with the electrolyte paste or gel. These types of sensors are more properly referred to as "silver/silver chloride" or Ag/AgCl sensors. Due to their low cost and more ready availability, Ag/AgCl sensors are being used more widely in many applications.

EEG Sensors

- Sensor type—gold, silver, silver-chloride, tin, etc.
- Sensor location—at least one sensor placed on scalp.
- Sensor attachment—requires electrolyte paste, gel, or solution.
- Maintain an electrically secure connection.

Sensor Types

- Disposable (gel-less and pre-gelled).
- Reusable disc sensors (gold or silver).
- Reusable sensor assemblies.
- Headbands, hats, etc.
- Saline-based electrodes—sodium chloride or potassium chloride.

EEG Principles

- Sensors pick up skin potential.
- Amplifiers create difference signal from each pair of sensors.
- Cannot measure "one" sensor, only a pair.
- Three leads per channel—active, reference, ground.
- Each channel yields a signal consisting of microvolts varying in time.

4

EEG DIGITIZATION
AND PROCESSING

When working with the digital EEG, it is important to keep several distinctions clear. One is that any abstraction of the EEG wave into a measure, referred to here as a "metric," involves assumptions and compromises. Another is that there is no "correct" way to approach EEG quantification. Opinions and preferences must be tempered with clinical experience and practical decisions that place the client's outcome at the forefront. There are many ways to reduce EEG waveforms to numbers, and it is essential to be precise about what is being monitored, assessed, or trained. It should also be noted that there are strong opinions and biases with regard to these choices. For example, some practitioners swear by raw power and will only use relative power under certain circumstances. Other clinicians will use relative power only and distrust raw power. Still others will say that power is not a useful measure at all and insist on using only amplitude.

Figure 4.1 illustrates a simple sinewave ("sinusoidal") signal. The basic properties of a repetitive signal are its peak and trough amplitudes, as well as its cycle length, also referred to as its wavelength. The frequency is the inverse of the wavelength, and is expressed in cycles per second, or hertz. Fundamentally, amplitude is a measure of how large a signal is, and is generally expressed in microvolts. Strictly speaking, amplitude is the momentary value of the waveform at any instant. Thus, it changes with every sample, and is a dynamic measurement. Generally, however, when speaking of amplitude, practitioners are actually referring to "magnitude," which is the value of the signal as a general property, such as its peak-to-peak size or its root-mean-square value. Figure 4.2 shows the relationship between amplitude and magnitude, and also shows the raw signal along with a filtered signal.

Figure 4.3 shows the variation in a signal's amplitude and frequency, illustrating that they can vary independently.

Peak-to-peak (P-P) and root-mean-square (RMS) are two ways to measure the magnitude of a signal. P-P comes more from the physiological world, while RMS comes from the communications engineering world.

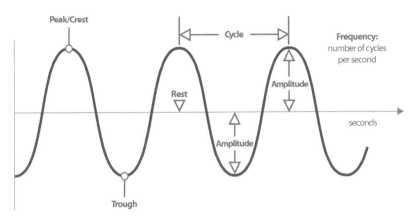

Figure 4.1 Basic properties of an oscillating signal.

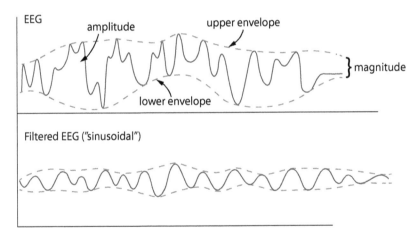

Figure 4.2 A complex signal shown along with its "envelope" (top) and a filtered signal, consisting of a narrow band of frequencies (bottom).

Both are still used in EEG and neurofeedback. Peak-to-peak is a measure of the excursion of the signal from its "bottom" to its "top." It is conceptually easy to understand, as it reflects the "height" of the waves on a screen. Root-mean-square, on the other hand, is a measure of the energy in the signal, and is derived from the amount of area under the waves themselves. Whereas P-P amplitude can be compared with height as a measure of an object, RMS magnitude is more like the weight of the object. Both are valid quantifications but they look at the signal differently. If the wave is purely sinusoidal, then there is a strict proportion between P-P and RMS, which is a ratio of 2.8 (twice the square root of 2, for mathematical reasons).

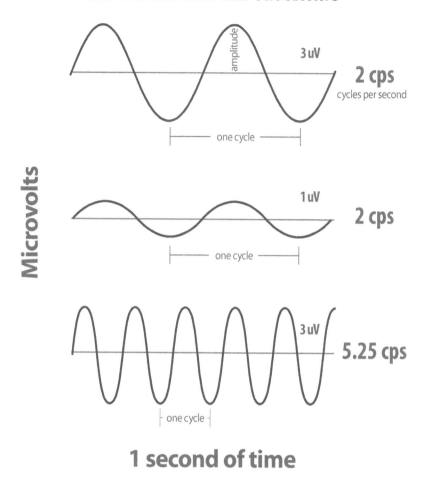

Figure 4.3 A signal that is slow (2 Hz) and large (3 microvolts) (top); a signal that is slow (2 Hz) and small (1 microvolt) (middle); a signal that is faster (5.25 Hz) and large (3 microvolts) (bottom).

When expressing EEG signal sizes, it is important to specify if it is P-P or RMS, as confusion can result if this is not made clear.

In addition to the amplitude or magnitude of an EEG signal, we can also express its frequency. Whereas amplitude is a measure of how large the signal is, frequency is a measure of how fast the signal is. No real signal actually consists of a single frequency, but we can identify the predominant frequency and express it in cycles per second, reflecting how fast the signal is oscillating. In addition to having amplitude and frequency, the EEG signal will typically vary in time in a manner we refer to as waxing and waning. In fact, this waxing and waning is visually distinct, and experienced EEG practitioners learn to recognize it.

In QEEG, and in neurofeedback, we try to reduce the signal to a frequency and amplitude so that we can work with it. In the case of QEEG, we typically obtain a long-term average of the signal, which provides a statistical measure of how the signal has behaved over a certain period of time. This is generally on the order of one minute or more, so that a considerable amount of information regarding the variation is lost in the QEEG analysis.

It also should be understood that the average amplitude or magnitude provided in a QEEG report reflects as much the time behavior and variation of the signal in time as it does the actual magnitude of the signal. For example, two individuals could have identical alpha waves, but in one person it is expressed 30 percent of the time, and, in the other, it is expressed 60 percent of the time. Therefore, the amplitude of the alpha wave in the second case would be reported as twice as large as in the first. However, the fact is not that the second person's alpha wave is any larger; it is simply that it is present twice as often, and this causes the average value to be twice as large.

When computing and reporting the frequency of an EEG signal, there are various means to achieve this measurement. When an FFT analysis is done, it is possible to identify a peak frequency and select it from the bins, typically with a 1 Hz resolution. When more precision is needed, it is possible to compute a mean frequency as a weighted average of this data.

Modern neurofeedback systems are based upon a computer implementation, most often a general-purpose personal computer (PC). Therefore, the principles of digital sampling and signal processing are applied, and these affect the system capabilities and limitations.

EEG Acquisition Parameters

- Digitization—converts from analog to digital.
- Sampling rate—how fast signal is sampled.
- Sampling resolution—how fine-grained.
- Processing model—spectral analysis or filtering, thresholding, displays, sound feedback, etc.
- Digital filters or similar algorithms selectively measure frequency information.
- Protocol processing via thresholds, etc.
- Computer produces graphics, sounds.

Principles of Sampling

Sampling Resolution

In order to reduce it to a digital form, a signal must be "sampled," which is to convert it into a number in the computer. The sampling accuracy, or resolution, are described in terms of the number of digital bits used to sample the signal. Typically, a minimum of 8 or 10 bits are used in the lowest-cost systems, 12 to 16 bits is more typical, and up to 24 bits are used in the highest-resolution systems. One significant benefit of 24-bit sampling is that it is possible to sample the entire range of the signal, including the DC component, and save it accurately. For example, a digitizer that uses 24 bits and has a resolution of 0.1 microvolts still has "headroom" of approximately 1 volt, providing excellent dynamic range. Systems with less than 24 bits must be AC-coupled to avoid the extremely large offset voltages that would take the signal outside the range of the digitizer.

Sampling Rate

The second major factor in sampling is the rate, in samples per second, that the signal is sampled at. In effect, the signal then becomes a chopped version of the original signal, which can introduce inaccuracy and distortion if it is not fast enough. In order to ensure that the frequencies are properly represented in an FFT-type analysis, the signal must be sampled at at least twice the highest frequency of interest. However, this rate does not ensure adequate visual representation of the signal, since it only guarantees two samples per cycle of the fastest frequency. Therefore, much higher sampling rates are used in QEEG and neurofeedback, typically 1,024 samples per second or greater. Higher sampling rates further ensure that the signal will

---

Frequency Analysis Using the FFT

- Fast Fourier Transform.
- Like a prism—breaks signal into bands.
- EEG data in "epochs"—chunks of time.
- Frequency in "bins" (e.g. 1 Hz, 2 Hz, etc.).
- Sees all frequencies at once.
- Sliding window in time.
- Accurate, but delay due to epoch length.
- Useful for percent energy, spectral correlation.
- Generally accepted for assessment purposes.

not be contaminated by harmonics of the power line noise, which can themselves extend to hundreds of hertz.

The Fast Fourier Transform (FFT) is the most common method of QEEG analysis, and forms the basis of many advanced methods. The FFT is simply a fast version of the Fourier Transform, which is a mathematical procedure developed in the 1850s by Joseph Fourier. While the FFT provides certain efficiencies in computer resources, it does not overcome any of the limitations of sampling rate or epoch size that are discussed below.

The Fourier Transform consists of an operation that multiplies a signal by a sinewave at some frequency and a cosine wave at the same frequency. These two results are averaged over time, and combined to produce an estimate of the power and phase of the signal.

Window (Epoch) Size and Frequency Resolution

When performing an FFT analysis, the sampled signal is further broken, into "epochs" which are of finite size, typically one or two seconds. The window (or epoch) size is an important factor in FFT analysis. It determines the lowest frequency that can be distinguished by mathematical analysis. The step, or "bin," size of the FFT is dictated by the epoch size. This frequency is equal to the inverse of the epoch size. Therefore, a one-second epoch will provide FFT frequency bins of 1, 2, 3, . . . Hz. The highest frequency is determined as ½ of the sampling rate. Therefore, if a signal is sampled at 256 samples per second, the highest frequency of analysis would be 128 Hz.

The limitations of sampling rate and epoch length are absolute, and are based upon mathematical principles. For example, if one wishes to have an FFT frequency resolution of ⅒ Hz, it is necessary to use a 10-second epoch size. This, in turn, limits the responsiveness of the system, since 10 seconds of EEG are taken into account when calculating parameters.

Fourier Transform

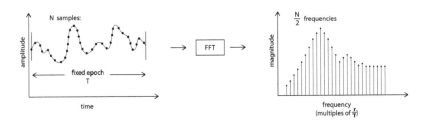

Figure 4.4 Illustrating the use of the Fourier Transform to convert a time-domain signal into its frequency components.

Frequency Aliasing and Leakage

Several types of distortion and error can occur with any FFT or similar digitally sampled and epoch-based analysis. One type of distortion is aliasing, which occurs when there is a signal that is faster than ½ the sampling rate. For example, if an EEG signal is sampled at 256 samples per second and there is a harmonic of the 60 Hz power line at the fourth harmonic (240 Hz), this will show up as a 16 Hz signal that is not due to the EEG, but is due to the noise artifact. Due to the presence of harmonics of line artifacts, QEEG systems typically operate at 512, 1024, or more samples per second to avoid the aliasing of power line harmonic noise.

Leakage is another form of artifact that occurs when the edges of the sampling epoch are not smooth. That is, if the signal has a nonzero value at the edges of the boundary, then false frequencies will appear in the FFT result. This is because the fundamental assumption of the Fourier series is that the signal is repetitive, and cyclic. This effect is called leakage, or the "Gibbs" effect. When the mathematics stitches the epochs together, additional frequencies are introduced. In order to avoid leakage, the data in the epoch must be "tapered" with a function that brings it to zero at the edges. One result is that the signals of interest must be in the center of the epoch window in order to be reflected in the analysis. This produces an intrinsic delay in FFT-based systems, regardless of the speed of the computer. Also, it is typical to not compute the FFT every time a new data point is sampled, but to wait for a certain amount of data. For example, a one-second FFT could be computed eight times per second by sliding the EEG data 125 milliseconds each time and recomputing the FFT. Thus, as features of interest slide into the center of the epoch, they will show up in the data.

The FFT suffers from several computational limitations that must be considered. First, it is necessary to choose an epoch size, generally one or two seconds in length. This is the length of the input signal that is analyzed in one chunk to gather the frequency estimates. The bin size will equal the inverse of the epoch size. Thus, a one-second epoch will result in 1 Hz bins.

The sampling rate also comes into play in the FFT. The sampling rate dictates the number of times the signal can be divided into pieces to provide all the bins. The maximum frequency that can be estimated is equal to ½ of the sampling rate. Thus, if a signal is recorded at 240 samples per second, the resulting FFT would have its highest bins set at a maximum frequency of 120 Hz.

When the FFT is applied, the epoch is generally windowed by applying a smoothing function that makes the signal close to zero at the beginning and end of the epoch. As a result of this windowing, the FFT is unable to show a component unless it is roughly in the middle of the epoch. Thus, if a one-second epoch is used, there is a built-in delay of ½ second for any component to be readily visible. This delay is generally considered unacceptable for real-time feedback.

JTFA

One method that overcomes the limitations of FFT epoch size is that of joint time-frequency analysis (JTFA). This method is similar to the FFT in that it uses sines and cosines, but it does not use a fixed epoch size. Instead, the intermediate results are passed through a low-pass filter that produces a slowed-down estimate of the frequency content, but does not require the signal to slide into a fixed epoch. Rather, data can be computed on every data point, providing rapid estimates of changes in EEG.

Digital Filtering

- Mathematical processing in real time.
- Continuous data analysis.
- Point-by-point results.
- Any frequency bands possible.
- Many types of filters possible.
- Generally fast response, restricted to defined bandwidth.
- Bandpass filter is like a colored glass.
- Passes only the frequencies designated.
- Separate components by bands.
- Frequency response (bandwidth and center frequency).
- Time response (time constant and "resonance").

Summary—FFT Versus JTFA

- FFT emphasizes the data in the middle of the epoch.
- JTFA emphasizes the most recent data.
- FFT is computed on each epoch, typically up to eight times per second.
- JTFA is computed on every data point, typically up to 256 times per second.
- FFT analyzes all frequency bins, like a prism.
- JTFA analyzes a preset frequency band, like a colored filter.

Digital Filters

Digital filtering is another approach to recovering EEG frequency-related information in real time. While there are various approaches to designing and implementing digital filters, they all share certain common strengths and weaknesses. Among their strengths is the ability to respond rapidly to sudden changes in EEG signals.

Figure 4.5 illustrates a signal being digitally filtered. One important factor with digital filters is that their bandwidth and frequency limits must be specified beforehand. In typical neural feedback systems, a minimum of three digital filters is generally provided, and eight or more such filters is becoming the norm. It is common to allow the user to select the filter type (Butterworth, Chebycheff, elliptical) and order (one, two, three up to 1,011 or 1,012). The choice of filter type and order, as well as the placement of corner frequencies, is a matter of significant personal preference and experience, as well as the application.

There are different biases with regard to digital filter design and use. Some practitioners tend to favor low-order filters because they offer the fastest response time. They also provide the least selectivity, but those who prefer them believe that the trainee's brain will sort through the information and reject what it deems not relevant. Low-order digital filters are best used when doing high-frequency training, such as SMR or beta, or with inexperienced clients or children.

Those who prefer high-order filters emphasize selectivity, and the ability to reject signals that are outside of the desired passband. High-order filters do require somewhat longer times to respond (a six order filter may require three cycles of the input signal). However, the benefits in terms of rejecting any out-of-band signals are considered of importance. In a general neural

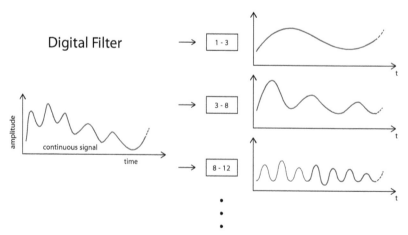

Figure 4.5 A raw signal with digitally filtered signals using various bandwidths.

feedback practice that serves a range of clients and concerns, it is likely that the practitioner will want to adjust filters based on the client and those factors that are considered of greatest priority.

The dynamics of filter response play an important role in neurofeedback. It is not generally possible to determine the important concerns from first principles alone, and the realities of the brain and EEG must also be taken into consideration. For example, alpha bursts are typically 100 to 500 milliseconds long, and the center frequency of the alpha wave is usually found in the range of 9 to 11 cycles per second. In order to adequately respond to the waxing and waning, a bandwidth of about 4 Hz is necessary, which is the primary reason that alpha filters are generally set at 8–12 Hz. SMR bursts are similar to alpha but slightly faster, typically centered at 14 Hz, and last from 80 to 200 milliseconds. Gamma, however, typically consists of very short bursts, as short as 20 to 50 milliseconds, and are therefore harder to see with a narrowband filter. In order to respond adequately to gamma bursting, a filter should be about 10 Hz wide (e.g. 35–45 Hz).

Filter Bandwidth, Type, and Order

When applying digital filters for neurofeedback, a different set of para-meters can be selected or adjusted. These choices will often depend on the particular situation, and cannot be dictated by general principles. A digital filter is defined by both its low and high cutoff frequencies, but also by its "order." Order is a measure of the sharpness of the cutoff region, in what is called the "stop band" of the filter. No realistic filter can entirely suppress all out-of-band signals due to mathematical limitations. In principle, an infinitely sharp filter could exist, but it would take forever to respond, and would have to look into the past, as well as into the future.

There are important tradeoffs in digital filter design and use that are insurmountable, even in principle. One tradeoff is that between filter order and response time. Put simply, the more sharply a filter cuts off the unwanted frequencies, the longer it will take to respond to a change in the input. A similar consideration is the fact that filter response time is also inversely proportional to the filter bandwidth. The reader may have noticed that the bandwidths defined for higher-frequency complements tend to be wider than those for lower-frequency complements. One important reality is that the low-frequency complements, such as alpha or theta, wax and wane much more slowly than higher-frequency complements. While an alpha outburst may easily last 500 ms or more, a data burst will rarely be longer than 100 ms. Therefore, if a filter is to show a brief burst of beta, then it must have a wider bandwidth, up to 10 Hz, in order to respond quickly enough. As an example, when measuring gamma, it is common to set the filter limits at 35 Hz and 45 Hz, not because the gamma rhythm is in and in determined that frequency in this range, but because the filter must be able to reflect short bursts.

Filter Order

- Describes slope of "reject" area outside of main passband.
- Low order = "shallow" skirts.
  - Faster, but less selective.
- High order = "steep" skirts.
  - Slower, but more selective.
- Typical values 2, 3, . . . 6 order filters.

Filter order is another important parameter, and it is set independently of the corner frequencies and bandwidth. Any filter order can be used with any bandwidth, and the choices are made on similar but slightly different criteria. Filter order reflects the amount of data that the filter processes, and it is reflected in how sharply the cutoff bands reduce out-of-band frequencies. The tradeoff is that the sharper the cutoff, the more cycles of data the filter needs in order to respond. This requirement causes higher-order filters to respond more slowly to changes in signals.

I once received a call from a client who said that his equipment was not showing gamma properly. I asked what his filter settings were, and he said 40 Hz. When I asked what the low frequency setting was, he said 40 Hz. When I asked what the high frequency setting was, he said 40 Hz. He had set his filter at 40 Hz with a bandwidth of 0 Hz. Given that this filter had zero bandwidth, there was no way it could respond to anything at all. I instructed him to set his gamma filter at 35–45 Hz and to use a low-filter order, such as 1 or 2. With these changes, he was able to measure gamma bursts quite readily.

Filter Order Recommendations

- Low order (typically 2, 3):
  High-frequency training—SMR, beta, gamma.
  Beginners, children, peak performance.
  Response has more "pop," picks up short bursts.
- High order (typically 5, 6):
  Low frequency training—theta, alpha.
  Advanced, adults, meditation.
  Response is more accurate, requires longer bursts.

Quadrature Filter

The quadrature filter (or "modulating filter" or "Weaver filter") is an approach to filter design that combines the strengths of FFT/JTFA and digital filtering. It provides filtering with readily adjustable center frequency and independently adjustable filter bandpass characteristics. It consists of a front end that multiplies by sines and cosines like a JTFA, and filters the signal with specifically tailored low-pass filters. The resulting complex coefficients are then combined in such a way as to provide the filtered waveform, along with its envelope value, as direct computations (Collura, 1990). It is thus superior to FFT or JTFA in that it produces phase-sensitive time-domain signals in real time, and it is superior to digital filtering in that the envelope and phase information are computed directly, and does not have to be extracted from a waveform. This approach also provides perfectly symmetrical passbands and the ability to place the center frequency with extreme precision. With a quadrature filter, establishing a precise filter at 12.55 Hz, for example, with a bandwidth of 2.46 Hz, is a simple matter, whereas a traditional filter with these properties would have to be designed for each specific combination of settings. The quadrature filter also has guaranteed zero phase delay at the center of the passband. The resulting complex data can be readily adapted to real-time calculations, such as coherence, spectral correlations, or comodulation. It is thus well suited to connectivity-based neurofeedback systems.

There is an important distinction to be made when interpreting EEG power data using retrospective analysis. When an average value of alpha of eight microvolts is reported for a one-minute interval, this means the average value over that minute is eight microvolts at any given instant, and the amplitude might be as low as 1 and as large as 15 or even 20. Therefore, the average value is as much an indicator of what is happening in time as it is the size of individual alpha bursts.

A trainee could increase his or her alpha in a feedback task not by making alpha bursts any larger, but simply by making them either more frequent or longer in duration. Therefore EEG operant training can be viewed in a context that emphasizes behavior in time rather than extent of any given amplitude. Therefore, increasing alpha in a neural feedback task does not mean to make alpha bigger; it means to make it more often.

This understanding that EEG magnitudes reflect time the behavior is important when interpreting results of operant training. A client whose task is to increase a given complement can understand that the issue is not so much one of trying or of making something large through effort. Rather, the task is one of allowing the event to occur more frequently and learning the internal states associated with the increased occurrence of the rewarded complement.

This understanding is also important when designing neural feedback protocols. We shall see that flexibility is a key issue. Therefore, if a client presents with low alpha, say four microvolts, this means primarily that the client has fewer occurrences of alpha bursts, not necessarily that his or her alpha waves are smaller. What is needed in this case is increased flexibility, so that the brain spends more time at larger amplitudes. However, the goal is not necessarily that the EEG alpha goes to a normal value, say eight microvolts, and sits there, and alpha, which is nonvarying, is abnormal, regardless of its value.

The importance of the short-term dynamics of the EEG is another reason why visual inspection of EEG waves is important. QEEG analysis tends to obscure short-term variations and hide them behind statistics and static maps. A well-designed neurofeedback practice will generally incorporate visual inspection of EEG waveforms and interpretation of QEEG data in the context of where the brain may be stuck and where additional flexibility (and appropriateness) are indicated.

The importance of EEG time dynamics is also reflected in the use of training parameters, such as sustained reward criterion (SRC), refractory period, and averaging windows or damping factors. These factors all provide ways to adjust the system response to facilitate learning. Based upon the principles of operant conditioning, the organism, which is the brain, must be provided with information that is timely, meaningful, and consistent.

The sustained reward criterion (SRC) is used to ensure that the training conditions have been met for a minimum period of time before a reward is issued. This is done to prevent spurious feedback and to ensure that the brain has actually produced lower rhythm. This would tend to avoid feedback based on values produced by noise or brief of sense. The refractory period (RP) is introduced to allow the organism to consolidate the learning associated with each reward. If rewards are issued to rapidly, learning is compromised because the consolidation period is interrupted. This consolidation is associated with the post-reinforcement synchronization (PRS) described previously.

Sustained Reward Criterion

The SRC is a duration of time that the event condition must be held for before the event becomes "true." It can be used to ensure that the event conditions are true continuously for a minimum time, before the event action is taken, and the event flag is set to "true." It is managed continuously in the following manner. The following steps are taken on a continuous basis, at a rate of approximately 30 times per second:

1. If the event condition is true, the amount of time credited toward the SRC is increased.
2. If the SRC duration has been met, the event is set to true, the amount of time toward the SRC is reset to zero, and the refractory period begins.

The RP is a duration of time after an event becomes true when two things happen:

1. The event remains "true" during the RP.
2. No conditions are tested during this period. Therefore, after the RP time has elapsed, the system again starts to count up, from zero, the time that the event condition is met in order to meet the SRC.

Refractory Period

Note that, during the RP, the trainee cannot accumulate any credits toward the next reward. It is only after the RP has elapsed that the checking of the event condition again resumes. This should become clear in the examples given below. If both the SRC and RP are set to zero, the system behaves normally. The event becomes "true" the instant that the condition is met, and will become "false" the instant that the condition is not met.

If the SRC is set to a value, and the RP is zero, then the event will become true only after the condition has been met for a period of time equal to the SRC. It will then immediately become false again until the SRC is again met. If, for example, the event condition is continually met, this will produce brief instants of the event being true, separated by intervals equal to the SRC.

If the SRC is zero, and the RP is set to a value, then the event will become true the instant that the condition is met. It will then remain true for a period of time equal to the RP, after which it will become false. It will immediately then become possible for the event to become true if the condition is met. If the event condition is continually met, this will produce periods of the event being true, separated by brief instants of it being false.

Color Plate 6 shows typical operation. In this example, the variable being fed back is the coherence, which will be explained in detail in Chapter 6. The top panel shows the raw coherence values and the coherence threshold for alpha. The second panel shows the coherence and coherence threshold on a scrolling trend graph. The third panel shows the flag for event 1, showing the times of it being true (value 1) and false (value 0). Note that the times of being true are, in this example, always 1,000 milliseconds long. Note also that the event does not become true until the coherence has been above threshold for 1,000 milliseconds.

Color Plate 7 shows a complex protocol in operation, with an animation and a game screen working alongside. Both the animation and the game advance during the refractory period. Thus, one-second bursts of game or animation are provided after the sustained reward criterion is satisfied. It is also possible to configure the video player to play one frame of an animation for each reward, which would occur at the beginning of the refractory period immediately after the SRC is satisfied.

Note that if a sustained voice is chosen, it will be heard during the entire RP. If a percussive voice is used, the trainee will hear one brief tone, then silence during the refractory period. The games and animations all progress during the RP. It should be further noted that averaging windows or damping factors can also be introduced in order to stabilize system response. Specific times and factors used are issues of clinical art, and particular settings may be unique to particular developers.

5

EEG COMPONENTS AND
THEIR PROPERTIES

The EEG typically consists of a complex waveform that includes a mixture of frequencies. However, two considerations motivate us to identify specific components. The first is that often a particular type of wave dominates, and is visually prominent. When this occurs, we say that the EEG is in that particular state, such as "in delta" or "in theta." The second consideration is that when frequency transforms or filters are used, it is possible to isolate a component band, even in the presence of other components. Therefore, regardless of which rhythms are dominant, if any, we can always identify component bands using computer processing.

I prefer to refer to these EEG components as "component bands" rather than "frequencies" or "bandwidths." This is because they are distinguished more properly by when and where they occur in the brain, their visual appearance, and their physiological meaning. The use of frequencies to distinguish them is rather artificial, and can lead to some ambiguities. A particular component may appear outside of its customary frequency range, and just because an EEG component is in a particular range does not mean that it necessarily conforms to that band's usual definition. For example, alpha may be less than 8 or more than 12, while still meeting the definition of alpha. It should also be emphasized that components are often not truly "sinusoidal" in appearance, and have distinctive morphology. Frequency

---

Typical EEG Component Band Ranges

- Delta 1–3 Hz
- Theta 4–7 Hz
- Alpha 8–12 Hz
- Low beta 12–15 Hz (SMR)
- Beta 15–20 Hz
- High beta 20–35 Hz (may contain EMG)
- Gamma 40 Hz

---

analysis, such as the Fourier Transform, assumes that waves are pure sine-waves. Any deviation from a pure sinewave leads to the appearance of higher harmonics, thus complicating the mathematical analysis. Therefore, a visual inspection of the EEG is always important to avoid these concerns.

It should be emphasized at the outset that the common EEG components are defined not by their exact frequency bands, but by their properties in terms of distribution in time and space, relationship to physiological states, and other properties. The primary EEG complements have been identified through clinical and research experience, and the associated frequency ranges have come along afterward. The frequency bands, therefore, describe the complements but do not define them. EEG complements can and do exist outside of their defined ranges, and it is also true that more than one complement may exist in a given frequency band range. Therefore, it is important not to arbitrarily identify any EEG rhythm based solely on its apparent frequency. The location and behavior of the complement are also important, as is the state of the client, possible medications, drowsiness, and other factors.

Delta is the slowest of the rhythmic EEG complements and is generally considered to be between 1 and 3 or 4 Hz. Upon visual inspection, delta is rarely, if ever, sinusoidal. Rather, it tends to have a distinctive wandering pattern and its shape (morphology) is important in assigning its origins. A small amount of delta is normal. However, excess delta may appear either focally or globally. Focal excess delta is associated with localized injury or insult, while global delta excess suggests toxicity, generalized pathology, aging, or other systemic issues. As it generally reflects injury or dysfunction, excess focal delta is often associated with lack of function in the affected areas. In such cases, downtraining the excess delta is often the indicated option. Downtraining of delta generally has the effect of reactivating the involved areas by rewarding for desynchronization, which produces higher frequencies.

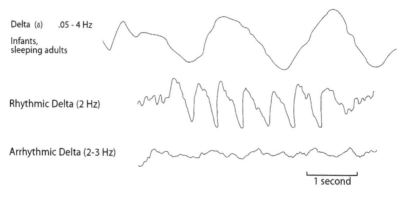

Delta (δ)   .05 - 4 Hz
Infants,
sleeping adults

Rhythmic Delta (2 Hz)

Arrhythmic Delta (2-3 Hz)

1 second

Figure 5.1 Examples of various forms of delta waves.

Delta (0.05–4 Hz)

- Distribution: broad, diffused, bilateral, widespread.
- Pathology: trauma, toxicity, neuropathy.
- Subjective states: deep, dreamless sleep, trance, unconscious.
- Tasks and behaviors: lethargic, not attentive.
- Physiological correlates: not moving, low-level arousal.
- Training effects: drowsiness, trance, deeply relaxed.

Theta is a rhythm that is mediated by subthalamic mechanisms, and, like delta, tends to have a distinctive non-sinusoidal appearance. A certain amount of theta is normal, particularly in the frontal areas, where it can be associated with a volition and movement. However, access theta is among the most common deviations associated with brain dysregulation. Focal theta is often seen in regions that are "off line" and theta downtraining is among the most common options when this is evident.

Despite the association of theta with inattention and internalized thought, it should be recognized that theta is also associated with creative thoughts and memory retrieval. Therefore, because it may occur at moderate levels even in a waking brain, it should not be regarded as an intrinsically "bad" rhythm that always needs to be minimized. Rather, the emphasis is on flexibility and appropriateness.

Theta (Typically 4–7 Hz)

- Low-frequency rhythm associated with internalized thoughts.
- Mediated by subthalamic mechanisms.
- Associated with memory consolidation.
- Generally non-sinusoidal, irregular.
- Seen during hypnogogic reverie.
- Seen as precursor and sequel to sleep.
- Edison's "creativity" state.
- Distribution: regional, many lobes, laterlized or diffuse.
- Subjective states: intuitive, creative, recall, fantasy, imagery, dreamlike.
- Tasks and behavior: creative, but may be distracted, unfocussed.
- Physiological correlates: healing, integration of mind and body.
- Effects: enhanced, drifting, trancelike, suppressed, concentration, focus.

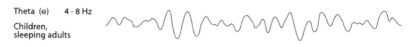

Theta (θ)   4 - 8 Hz

Children,
sleeping adults

Figure 5.2 Example of theta waves.

The alpha wave is sometimes defined as the "8–12 Hz" rhythm. However, this factor is only incidental in what distinguishes the alpha rhythm. The key aspects of the alpha rhythm is that it is a resting rhythm of the visual system, that it is maximum posteriorly, that it increases when the eyes close, and that it is symmetrical with a characteristic waxing and waning. All of these factors stem from the fact that it is a thalamo-cortical reverberation involving the visual pathways and the primary visual cortex, and that it represents the visual system relaxing and also performing some types of background memory scanning. An individual is also typically aware, but relaxed, during periods of alpha.

The actual frequency of alpha can vary outside the 8–12 Hz range, and other components can also show up in this range. Therefore, any signal that is in the 8–12 Hz range is not necessarily alpha. What is certain is that if one sees a signal that is sinusoidal and symmetrical, has a characteristic waxing and waning, is maximum posteriorly, and increases when the eyes closed, then it is an alpha wave.

Figure 5.4 shows the typical range of alpha peak frequencies in a normal population. It should be noted that a significant percentage of the population will have a peak alpha frequency that is different from the typical value of 10 Hz.

Another rhythm that can occupy the alpha band but which is not alpha is the "mu" rhythm. This wave has a visually distinct "wicket" appearance, and is clearly non-sinusoidal. It also does not have a characteristic waxing and waning, and is more often maximum centrally, not occipitally. Its meaning is by no means as clear as that of alpha, and some controversy remains whether it is abnormal or normal, and what clinical determinations can be made in its presence.

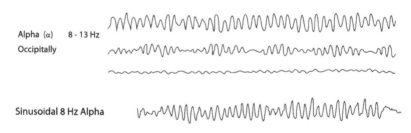

Alpha (α)   8 - 13 Hz

Occipitally

Sinusoidal 8 Hz Alpha

Figure 5.3 Alpha waves.

106

Alpha (Typically 8–12 Hz)

- Resting rhythm of the visual system.
- Increases when eyes are closed.
- Largest occipital—O1, O2.
- Characteristic waxing and waning.
- Generally sinusoidal, hemispheric symmetrical.
- Indicates relaxation.
- Role in background memory scanning.
- Round trip thalamus-cortex-thalamus ~100 ms.
- Typically 8–12 Hz, but may be 4–20 Hz.
- Distribution: regional, evolves entire lobes, strong occipital with closed eyes.
- Subjective states: relaxed, not drowsy.
- Tasks and behavior: meditation, no action.
- Physiological correlates: relaxed, healing.
- Effects: relaxation.

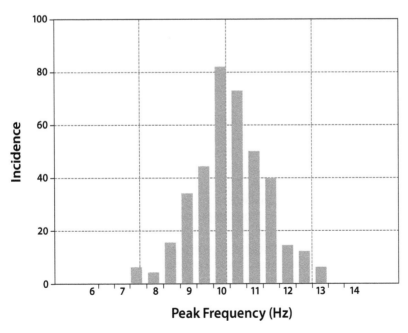

Figure 5.4 Typical range of alpha peak frequencies in a normal population.

Source: Data courtesy of David Kaiser (1994).

An interesting aspect of alpha biofeedback was revealed in a study reported by Plotkin and Rice (1981). In this study, a controlled experiment was devised in which half of the participants took part in alpha enhancement training and the other half took part in alpha reduction training. The expectation was that the alpha enhancement group would show improvement, while the alpha reduction group would not. What was discovered, however, was that both groups indicated improvements, including increased self-awareness and ability to relax. These investigators concluded that the alpha training experience was a placebo because of the similarity in results in both groups. However, a different interpretation is more likely. Whereas the alpha enhancement group indeed learned an alpha state, the other group was actually undergoing a form of activation training, or "squash" training. Interpreting this study as showing placebo effects is similar to having half of a group do pushups, and the other do pullups, and concluding that exercise is a placebo. Naively, these are opposite tasks, but, in reality, both are exercise. Similarly, both alpha enhancement and alpha reduction are beneficial neurofeedback tasks, and the presence of benefits in both groups does not imply that there is a placebo effect.

An important distinction must be made between *alpha* activity and *brain* activity in a brain region. Alpha activity is associated with reduced brain activation; when alpha waves are present, that location is in an idling state, and hence is less active. Therefore, when we see increased alpha waves, the brain is actually less active. An activated brain state is associated with high-frequency, low-amplitude EEG activity. This is the basis of the "squash" protocols, which will be discussed with training protocols. In essence, a training protocol that encourages the lowering of EEG amplitude, particularly alpha or theta amplitude, will result in an activation of the related brain areas.

Asymmetry of alpha, particularly frontal alpha, is important to mood. In normal individuals, left frontal alpha is typically 10 percent to 15 percent lower than right frontal alpha. This asymmetry is important for normal mood control. It has been reported (Baehr et al., 2001; Davidson and Begley, 2012) that depression is associated with higher left frontal alpha, and that operant training to restore the asymmetry in the direction of lower left frontal alpha results in mood improvement. The rationale behind this approach is the observation that the left frontal area is responsible for positive judgments and associated approach behavior, while the right frontal area mediates negative judgments and associated withdrawal behavior. For normal mood, the negative area (right side) should be somewhat less active than the positive area (left side). Therefore, a slightly lower alpha on the left corresponds with greater activation of this positive judgment area. Baehr et al. (2001) treated depressed clients with alpha lowering training on the left. Hammond (2005) demonstrated improvements in clients treated with a protocol that increased beta in the left frontal region.

Another important subtlety with regard to alpha is the presence of two basically different alpha ranges. The fast alpha range, between 10 and 12 Hz, is the typical occipital resting rhythm. It reflects background memory processing and an idle, yet not inattentive, state. The slow alpha, typically taken as 8–10 Hz, appears more frontally and is more associated with emotional processing. When EEG spectral displays are seen in real time, the independent waxing and waning of these two alphas is clearly evident. When performing assessments and neurofeedback training, it is becoming more common to distinguish between these two alpha bands, and to treat them individually. It is interesting in this regard to note that alpha may slow down with age. While significant alpha slowing is associated with degraded mental processing, a general slowing down with age may indicate that more processing is occurring at the endpoints of the thalamo-cortical cycling, thus delaying the cycle time and reducing the frequency. As seen in experienced meditators, for example, in this context, slowed alpha may indeed be an indicator of acquired knowledge, and possibly even wisdom.

Low beta is one of the more interesting brain rhythms, partially because it comprises the sensorimotor rhythm, when it is observed from the sensorimotor cortex. Low beta is actually an alpha wave if one considers that it is thalamo-cortical reverberation, and that it represents an idle state. Barry Sterman conditioned SMR in cats, and reported that cats that were trained to produce SMR were significantly more resistant to the adverse effects of a toxin (monomethyl hydrazine).

Sterman identified SMR as a resting rhythm of the motor system, and described it as indicating the intention to remain still. This is one of the more philosophically profound aspects of neural feedback: that it can indicate and train something as seemingly obscure as intention. Sterman initially began to operably train the SMR rhythm in cats after observing that they produced this rhythm when they were still. By using a reward consisting of broth and milk, he successfully trained some of the cats to increase their SMR rhythm. Later, fate intervened when these cats were randomly assigned to trials of withstanding toxic doses of monomethyl-hydrazine fuel. This later research was intended to assess the toxicity of this aviation fuel. However, anomalous results caused Sterman to reinvestigate the data. He then discovered that the operably trained cats were significantly more resistant to the toxic affects of the fuel. In essence, the SMR training had rendered the cats more resistant to the toxic challenge.

Sterman further observed that the operably trained cats were significantly more resistant to seizures. This led to investigations of SMR training as a means to reduce seizures in children. Overall, SMR training has emerged as a significant benefit in a wide range of situations, particularly related to pediatric attention and seizures, as well as helping in cases of insomnia. It appears that SMR training is a core mechanism associated with brain and body stability and resistance to stress.

13 Hz Spindles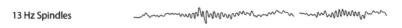

Figure 5.5 Examples of low beta or sensorimotor rhythm (SMR) at 13 Hz.

In the broad context, given that we have the ability to operatively condition a rhythm associated with the intention to remain still, as well as brain and body resilience, we can understand why SMR training has the clinical importance that has been seen over the last several decades. Rather than addressing behavioral issues, or using approaches that focus on symptoms, neural feedback of SMR, when applied to hyperactivity, gives clinicians a way to fundamentally alter a client's ability to be comfortable with stillness, in contrast to continually seeking stimulation and action.

Low Beta

- Distribution: localized by side and lobe.
- Subjective states: relaxed, focused, integrated.
- Tasks and behavior: relaxed, attentive.
- Physiological correlates: inhibited motion (when at sensorimotor cortex).
- Effects: relaxed focus, improved attentive ability.

Sensorimotor Rhythm (SMR)

- Resting rhythm of the motor system.
- Largest when body is inactive.
- Indicates intention not to move.
- Measured over sensorimotor strip C3/Cz/C4.
- Round-trip thalamus-cortex-thalamus ~80 ms.
- Typically 12–15 Hz.
- Also called "14 Hz" or "Tansey" rhythm.

Beta waves are those most generally associated with conscious, deliberate thought. When present, they indicate brain activation, and cortico-cortical communication. Because the cortico-cortical connections mediating beta tend to be between nearby sites ("short-range connections"), beta tends to be more localized than lower-frequency rhythms.

Beta is one of the more common complements trained in neurofeedback, and it is used as a way to train activation of specific areas. In particular, when beta deficits are evident, and clinical signs include those associated with under activation, beta training can be an effective way to activate the affected regions, and achieve more normalized thoughts and behavior. Beta is also used in peak performance training, in which clients without clinical complaints seek improved mental sharpness or acuity.

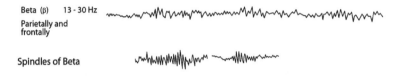

Beta (β)   13 - 30 Hz
Parietally and
frontally

Spindles of Beta

Figure 5.6 Examples of beta waves.

Case Report—Uptraining Right Frontal Beta?

A mother called to report that her son had reacted adversely to neurofeedback training. When questioned, she reported that she was uptraining beta on the right frontal area based on advice she had received on the internet. When asked why she was doing this, she replied that the EEG said that the boy did not have enough beta on the right front. When asked whether this was in absolute or relative power, she stated that she did not know. When asked if she knew what activation of the right frontal area would do, she said no. When she was informed that right frontal activation could precipitate negative behavior, she reported that that was what had just happened. What was happening in this case was that the boy had underactivated frontal areas, reflecting his general attentional problems. As a result, there were excessive low frequencies (theta and alpha) in this region. When the EEG was evaluated, one of the findings was that, in relative terms, the frontal areas had "too little beta." The beta was being compared to the excess slow activity, resulting in this judgment. However, taking this information and deciding to do beta uptraining on the right frontal area as a result, was a mistake. The correct path would have been to activate the left frontal area, in the form of downtraining theta or alpha, and allowing this to help improve mood, without overactivating the right frontal lobe.

Beta (Typically 15–20 Hz)

- Distribution: localized, over various areas.
- Subjective states: thinking, aware of self and surroundings.
- Tasks and behavior: mental activity.
- Physiological correlates: alert, active.
- Effects: increase mental ability, focus, alertness.

High Beta (Typically 20–30 Hz)

- Distribution: localized, very focused.
- Subjective states: alertness, agitation.
- Tasks and behavior: mental activities (math, planning, etc.).
- Physiological correlates: activation of mind and body functions.
- Effects: alertness, agitation.

Gamma (35–45 Hz)

- Also known as "Sheer" rhythm.
- Associated with cognitive binding.
- Collura (1987) and Collura et al. (2004) reported on 6–7 bursts per second in PSI states using FFT technique.
- Lutz et al. (2004) found sustained gamma in advanced meditators.
- Short bursts require wide (35–45 Hz) filters to detect.
- Others define:
    - 25–30 Hz (Thatcher and Lubar, 2009).
    - 32–64 Hz (Thornton and Carmody, 2009).
- Distribution: very localized.
- Subjective states: thinking, integrated thoughts.
- Tasks and behavior: high-level information processing "binding."
- Physiological correlates: information-rich tasks, integration of new material.
- Effects: improved mental clarity, efficiency, language facility.

There is evidence that the gamma rhythm is connected with low-frequency rhythms, such as theta, and that there may be a "gating" mechanism. The gamma bursts can appear as individual wavelets that occur at a low frequency rate and are relatively short. Collura (1987) and Collura et al. (2004) identified spectral signatures that suggested that bursts of 40 Hz activity at a rate of 6–7 per second in a clairvoyant subject, during successful trials, as distinguished from unsuccessful trials. Freeman et al. (2003) demonstrated phase resetting of the gamma rhythms, at rates of 7–9 per second. Lutz et al. (2004) also demonstrated enhanced gamma in experienced meditators.

Figure 5.7 shows the correlation between infra-slow (0.002–0.05) oscillations and conventional component bands. It is evident that, in addition to the expected correlation with delta and theta, there is a correlation with the variations in the gamma band as well.

Note that the shortness of the gamma bursts accounts for the fact that a wide filter bandwidth is required to track these events. The sidebands created by the modulation of the gamma bursts produces energy as far as 5 or more Hz away from the 40 Hz "carrier" band, so that the actual energy in the signal extends from 35 Hz to 45 Hz, at a minimum.

DC and Slow Cortical Potentials

DC and slow cortical potentials have been discussed in Chapter 2 in relation to neurofeedback mechanisms and training. It is sufficient to note here that

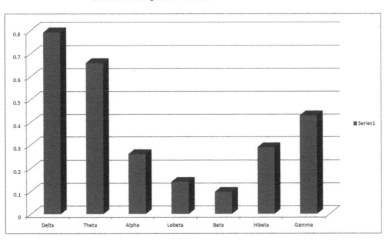

Figure 5.7 Correlation between infra-slow oscillations and conventional component bands.

the physiological mechanisms that generate the EEG operate at frequencies extending all the way down to the 0 Hz or "standing" potential.

DC (0–0.1 Hz)

- Standing potential, 0.0–1 Hz.
- Reflects glial, other mechanisms.
- Includes sensor offset and drift.
- May include "injury" potential.
- Difficult to record, may be unstable.
- Requires Ag/AgCl sensors.
- SCP is more useful clinically.

Slow cortical potentials consist of the signals that vary with long time-constants, moving above and below the baseline over periods of seconds. An SCP shift may occur over a period of one to five seconds, and reflects a change in cortical excitability.

SCP—Slow Cortical Potential

- Typically 0.01–2 Hz.
- May include glial origin.
- Associated with general brain activation.
- "Bareitschaft" potential evident preceding voluntary motor movement.
- Large shifts seen preceding seizures.
- Training useful in epilepsy, BCI.

Infra-Slow Potentials

A more recent development has been the use of feedback with filters set at very low frequencies. These are set so low that it no longer makes sense to think of the underlying signals as rhythms, but they take on the quality of shifts in the DC level, which may be thought of as transients. The lower a filter is set, the longer it takes to respond to a change in its input; correspondingly, the larger an input must be in order to register a change in the output.

The emerging use of feedback using very low frequencies has been referred to as "infra-low frequency" or "infra-slow fluctuation" potential work. Girten et al. (1973) observed such slow oscillations more than 40 years ago, but their use for neurofeedback has been relatively recent. The low-frequency cutoff can be set as low as 0.001 Hz, and frequency adjustments can be made with a resolution as low as 0.0001 Hz. This does not mean that the potentials oscillate with a period of $1/0.001 = 1,000$ seconds, which would be on the order of 16 minutes. Rather, the filters serve to block out all but the largest transient shifts in the DC baseline. Therefore, if filters are set, for example, with a range of from 0.001 to 0.0015 Hz, the low cutoff serves to bring the signal back to zero baseline with a very long time constant, and the high cutoff serves to ensure that only significant shifts in the baseline will be passed through the filters.

ILF (or ISF) work is generally done with the addition of inhibits on most, if not all, of the conventional EEG frequency bands. This changes the nature of the feedback so that there is general reinforcement when the EEG quiets in general, and additional rewards are provided when the DC level of the EEG shifts by a sufficient amount. It is possible to reward either positive or negative shifts separately, or to reward any shift.

Development of ILF/ISF neurofeedback has followed a primarily empirical path, with clinical experience and subjective reporting becoming a driving factor (Othmer and Othmer, 2008; Othmer, 2010). As a result, the scientific underpinnings and origins of these signals remain somewhat unclear and not without controversy. The factors that can potentially contribute to these fluctuations include both brain and non-brain sources, and influences including variations in skin and sensor properties cannot be discounted.

6

CONNECTIVITY-BASED
EEG BIOFEEDBACK

Once the EEG has been digitized and processed to extract relevant information, the question arises of how to produce useful metrics for assessment and training. It should be kept in mind that all computed metrics are the result of a conceptual and procedural process that involves certain assumptions. Based on these assumptions, a definition can be created, based upon which a measurement is defined, and then implemented via a computation. It should be emphasized that the result, a given "metric," has no absolute relationship to reality. Rather, its usefulness and applicability are subject to empirical validation. A variety of metrics have thus been created and applied, and yet there has been a limited uniform approach to understanding and evaluating them.

The use of connectivity introduces an entirely new dimension to neurofeedback. Training based upon amplitudes, powers, power ratios, or other metrics addresses cortical activation or relaxation. Any changes that result in communication or mutual activation will be secondary to this primary action. While changes in connectivity can, and surely do, occur even during power training, neurofeedback based upon connectivity has provided the ability to directly alter brain connections and how different regions of the brain interact. This has particular importance for issues such as attention, planning, perception, language, cognitive binding, and other high-level functions. For a more exhaustive review of these metrics and their properties, the reader is referred to Collura (2006). In this section, we look at the interpretation and use of various connectivity metrics in the realm of neurofeedback practice.

Coherence

The coherence measured between two signals is a concept derived from electrical and communication engineering (Carter, 1987). It is defined as the cross-spectrum normalized by the auto-spectra of the signals, and is a Pearson correlation coefficient in the complex domain.

116

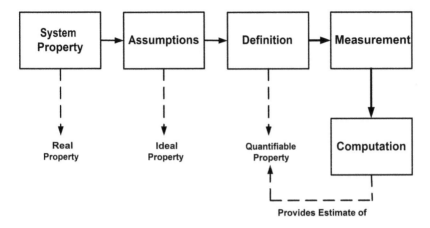

Figure 6.1 The path to defining a quantity or metric follows a series of steps, including identifying a system property, making assumptions, creating a definition, and then implementing the measurement and computing the relevant quantity.

Summary of Connectivity Measures

- Pure coherence (is relative phase stable?)
  - Do the sites share spectral energy?
  - Joint energy/sum of self-energy.
- Synchrony metric (phase and amplitude match?)
  - Do the waveforms rise and fall together?
  - Joint energy/sum of self-energy.
- Spectral correlation coefficient (are FFT amplitudes same?)
  - Are the sites similarly "tuned" in frequency?
  - Correlation (f) between amplitude spectra.
- Comodulation (components wax and wane together?)
  - Is there a time-relationship in activation patterns?
  - Correlation (t) between amplitude time-series.
- Phase (timing stable or same?)
  - Do the waveform peaks and valleys correlate?
  - Arctan of ratio of quadrature components.
- Sum/difference channels (direct comparison)
  - Do the waveforms line up by peaks and valleys?
  - Simply add or subtract raw waveforms.

$$\text{Coherence} = \frac{\left|H_{xy}\right|^2}{\left|H_{xx}\right|\left|H_{yy}\right|}$$

The numerator is the "cross-spectrum" or shared energy between the two signals, and the two terms in the denominator represent the "auto-spectra" or individual energies of the individual signals. The metric can be defined for any frequency component, or for a single FFT bin. It reflects the stability of the phase relationship between the signals and is independent of the signal amplitudes themselves. Coherence is a measure of the amount of information sharing between two sites. Technically, it is a measure of how stable the phase relationship is over time. If two sites consistently have a stable phase relationship, then they will have a high coherence. It should be evident that if two signals are highly coherent, then they also have to be at the same frequency. The peaks and valleys do not have to line up, however, to have a stable relationship.

Coherence is not intrinsically good or bad, and it should not be assumed that coherence should be particularly high or low for any given component or brain locations. As is typical in communication-based systems, the amount of connectivity must be appropriate and if it is either too large or too small can cause problems. David Kaiser (2008) has referred to this as a Goldilocks effect. This is one of the most important benefits of live z-score training. If a normative database is used that contains the normal ranges for coherence for different bands between different sites, then it becomes possible to train conductivity specifically within normative ranges, rather than simply up or down.

Analogies Regarding Coherence and Phase

Because coherence and phase are mathematical concepts, it can be difficult to explain them in simple terms. However, they are also dynamic system properties that reflect qualities that can be understood in other terms. We can use some analogies to help clarify key concepts.

Coherence is a measure of the amount of information shared at a given instant. Phase is a measure of the speed of information transfer at a given instant. We can use the analogy of a walkie-talkie as a medium that is fast and instantaneous but conveys relatively little information. This, therefore, has low coherence but small phase. As an alternative, a package of books would be transferred more slowly but conveys a large amount of information. This would have high coherence but large phase. There are times when a walkie-talkie is needed, such as to get someone's attention quickly. There are, however, also times when a package of books is appropriate, such as when learning a new topic. The brain, as a dynamical system, has both of these types of situations, and, therefore, the coherence

118

and phase observed in an EEG signal can vary widely in its connectivity, depending on the brain locations, frequencies, and tasks being monitored.

Hypo-coherence is a case in which information is not being shared. For example, two walkie-talkies that are turned off are an example of an extremely hypo-coherent situation. Hyper-coherence is the case in which a large amount of information is being shared between different brain locations. However, it should be kept in mind that this is not necessarily always a good thing. For example, if someone is watching TV intently, they are in a hyper-coherent relationship with the television. At the same time, however, they have a hypo-coherent relationship with anyone else in the room. Therefore, if communication with someone else in the room is important, this situation is not optimal.

In the brain, there are centers that need to be in communication, and there are also centers that, at times, need to be independent. High coherence implies high dependency, while low coherence implies low dependency. Therefore, low coherence can also be associated with differentiation or independence of functioning.

There are many clinically relevant situations in which coherence and phase abnormalities are important. And it is possible for either hyper-coherence or hypo-coherence to introduce a symptomatic deviation or a clinical concern. A hyper-coherent state may indicate excessive dependence between sites and a lack of differentiation. Therefore, hyper-coherence may, at times, be seen in clients with impaired cognitive abilities. Similarly, hypo-coherence indicates a lack of collective functioning, and the inability to distribute processing in the brain. Hypo-coherence is often seen in cases of attention or cognitive impairment as well. This is one reason that QEEG and neurofeedback have value in mental health work. Whereas two individuals may exhibit similar problems in their functioning, EEG can separate out different underlying causes and point the way for individualized assessment and treatment options.

It is important to note that the observation of high coherence between two sites does not necessarily imply that they are connected. For example, if a pair of sites are also in communication with a third location, which is serving as a source of information to both of them, then they will exhibit shared information. Often, the thalamus will be pacing more than one cortical area in a synchronized fashion so that coherence can be measured from and between the sites, although the relevant physical connectivities are the point-to-point connections between cortical locations and their respective thalamic projection nuclei. A real-world analogy would be a population watching or listening to a broadcast, which results in shared information between individuals who are not, in fact, in communication with each other. Coherence is, therefore, a neutral metric, in that it indicates shared information but provides no information relevant to why it is shared, how it is shared, or the direction of information flow.

Different levels of coherence and phase lead to different functional profiles. A hyper-coherent system, for example, has significant coordination but little differentiation. It is rather like having a baseball team with nine first basemen. A given task is very well executed but there is no opportunity for functional variation or flexibility. Similarly, a system with very low phase is very fast but may be too tightly coupled. Low phase indicates speed of communication, which would seem to be a universally good thing. However, in the brain, delays are required in order to process and integrate information, using the brain's considerable resources. If the process of integrating and evaluating information is cut short, decisions may be too fast and not optimal. Characteristics that might be anticipated in cases of highly phase-coupled individuals might include hyper-loquacity (excess, rambling speech), difficulty converging on logical conclusions, or issues with impulsivity. The individual who says "I knew as soon as I said it that it was wrong" is suffering from an inability to maintain appropriate connections and timing in service of anticipating the consequences of his or her actions (speech) and appropriately regulating his or her behavior.

The other extremes, those of hypo-coherence and excess phase, reflect a deficit in information sharing. Depending on the affected sites, different profiles may be anticipated. In the language system, excess phase delay may be associated with stuttering, word-grasping, or related language deficits. Low coherence, or excess phase delay, reflect an excess of differentiation. Functional sites that should work together are independent and, essentially, "doing their own thing" rather than participating in the coordinated effort. However, a long delay does not imply low coherence. A system may have a long delay but still exhibit high quality of information transfer, and thus high coherence. For example, if alpha from the anterior and posterior sites appears to be out of phase, but the phase delay is consistent, then the brain is still exhibiting high coherence in alpha. Or if one cortical area is in communication with another, but there is a regular processing delay, then coherence can still be high. A general analogy might be that if an individual receives his or her mail regularly the morning after it was sent, there is a delay of up to 24 hours, but a high amount of information involved in the transfer.

In order to estimate coherence in real time, a variation of joint time-frequency analysis may be used. This is compared with Fourier-based methods, or processing on the filtered waveforms, in Figure 6.2. Assessment techniques, and some real-time implementations, have used the Fourier Transform approach to compute connectivity metrics. This introduces computational delays associated with the use of finite-length epochs, as well as need to further average data to compute a valid correlation across time. The most direct and rapid method of computing real-time correlations such as coherence is to do the processing within the complex variables inside the joint time-frequency analysis. This provides a connectivity estimate that

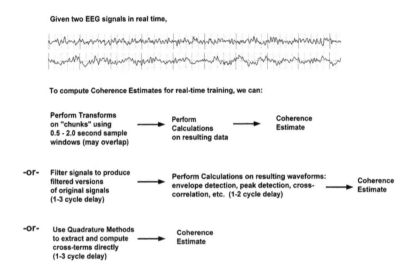

Figure 6.2 The processes by which coherence can be estimated in real time range from epoch or "chunk" oriented **FFT** or related transform methods, digital filtering, or quadrature methods. Of these, JTFA or quadrature methods provide the least computational delay due to signal processing steps.

can be computed on each data point and provide continual updating. This is also useful for estimating the time behavior of connectivity, such as the variability in coherence, which is an interesting metric.

Coherence basically asks "How stable is the phase relationship between two signals?" As can be seen in Figure 6.2, two channels of filtered alpha waves can be strongly correlated in this way. This reflects the underlying mechanism, which is a symmetric thalamo-cortical reverberation that is synchronized both at the thalamic and the cortical levels, producing the visible characteristic of peaks and valleys that are in a precise relationship between the two channels. See Color Plate 8.

Coherence

- Coherence reflects similarity between two channels.
- Measure of information sharing.
- Coherence may be trained up or down.
- "Goldilocks" effect—may be too high or too low at any given site.
- Alpha coherence can be trained up bilaterally (occipital or parietal) without adverse reaction.

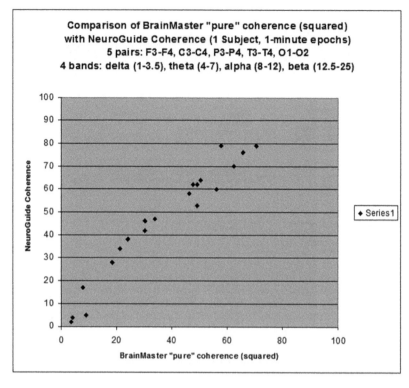

Figure 6.3 Agreement between two implementations of coherence, demonstrating match across four frequency bands and five sensor pairs, ranging from less than 2 percent to 80 percent coherence.

The question often arises regarding the match between different implementations of coherence or related metrics. It is true that such estimates depend strongly on certain parameter decisions and values, as well as details of the input signal. Figure 6.3 demonstrates the strong agreement that can be achieved when consistent methods are used (Collura, 2008).

Spectral Correlation Coefficient

Spectral correlation coefficient (SCC) is a metric that reflects how similar the activation patterns of two regions are. It is computed as a Pearson correlation between two sets of spectral arrays.

$$\text{Spectral correlation} = \frac{\left(\sum \left(|X_f||Y_f|\right)\right)}{\left(\sum |X_f|^2 \sum |Y_f|^2\right)}$$

SCC is expressed in percent, "where X and Y represent the Fourier magnitude series of the two channels" (Joffe, 1992). This is thus a measure of how similar the two signals' FFT spectra are in shape, regardless of phase, and independent of their absolute or relative magnitudes. It thus looks at whether the frequency distribution of the two sites is similar or not. In other words, if two regions have similar proportions of energy in the bands from 20 to 30 Hz, we would say that they have high SCC in beta. If the two have frequency distributions that look different, then the SCC would be low. Conceptually, if we appeal to the model that different cortical regions can facilitate communication by operating at similar frequencies, then this metric reflects that similarity. This can be thought of as the frequency of the "walkie-talkie" that each cortical region is operating. If two regions have a high SCC, then their walkie-talkies are operating on the same frequency bands. It thus reflects a potential for communication, as well as the likelihood that the regions might be working in concordance. See Color Plate 9.

Figure 6.4 shows the agreement between two implementations of SCC, showing the agreement across a range of frequency bands.

Spectral Correlation Coefficient (SCC)

- Measure of amplitude similarity in spectral energy—uses FFT amplitude data.
- Larger when two signals have similar power spectral shape.
- Completely ignores phase relationship.
- Meaningful for a single epoch.
- Random signals may have large correlation if spectra are similar.

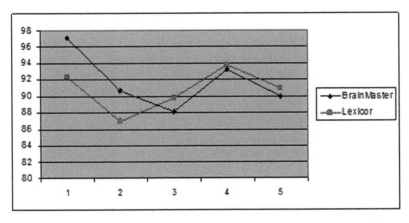

Figure 6.4 Match between two implementations of spectral correlation coefficient (SCC), showing match within 5 percent for five frequency bands (gamma, beta, alpha, theta, and delta).

Synchrony

Synchrony looks specifically at whether two signals have their peaks and valleys lined up. Synchrony is typified by the large, bilaterally symmetric alpha with eyes closed in a normal person. Synchrony is more generally used in peak performance contexts than in QEEG-based neural feedback. This is because synchrony is actually a special case of coherence. Whereas coherence looks at how stable the phase relationship is between two channels, synchrony looks at whether they are, in fact, in phase. Only a limited set of EEG complements and sites are generally truly synchronous, whereas normative values for coherence can be found between any pair of sites for any compound. The most common form of synchrony training for peak performance or mental fitness is alpha synchrony training. This can be done between two, three, or more sites. Whole-head alpha training in general, and synchrony in particular, are important modalities for mental fitness and clinical intervention, as typified by the work of Joe Kamiya, James V. Hardt, and Les Fehmi (Hardt and Kamiya, 1978; Fehmi and Robbins, 2007). See Color Plate 10.

Comodulation

Comodulation is also a Pearson correlation of the spectral energy in the EEG, but it looks across time rather than frequency.

$$\text{Comodulation} = \frac{\left(\sum\left(|X_t||Y_t|\right)\right)}{\left(\sum|X_t|^2 \sum|Y_t|^2\right)}$$

In this expression, the X and Y values represent successive measurements of the signal amplitudes across time for signals X and Y, respectively. At every instant at some sampling interval (typically eight per second), the amplitude of a given band is measured and put into an array over time. This sequence of amplitudes is then correlated with the sequence from other channels to see if they are related. A high comodulation indicates that the time patterns of the two sites are related in time. Typically, if they, in fact, rise and fall at the same time, they will have a high comodulation. However, the correlation can also be high if there is some delay between them, as long as the delay is consistent. For example, if every time one site produced a burst of beta and another site produced a burst 200 milliseconds later, this would show up as a high comodulation. To extend the walkie-talkie analogy above, the comodulation sees if the walkie-talkies are being turned on and off in a related fashion. This would again reflect the likelihood that the two sites are working together, or at least in a coordinated fashion.

It is evident that any of several mechanisms could result in comodulation, so its presence does not determine the mechanism, only the presence of a functional relationship. See Color Plate 11.

Comodulation

- Measures similarity in amplitudes across time—classically uses FFT amplitude data.
- Correlation between envelopes of two signals.
- Completely ignores phase relationship.
- Must be considered across time epoch.
- Reflects how similarly signals wax and wane together.
- Can be computed using digital filters.
- Random signals will have low comodulation.

Asymmetry

Asymmetry is not strictly a measure of connectivity, but it does reflect the mutual activation of different parts of the brain.

$$\text{Asymmetry} = \frac{A - B}{A + B}$$

Also, there are normative values of asymmetry that, if not met, can be reflected clinically. Asymmetry is simply the measure of the ratio of amplitude in any given band between two sites. One might naively assume that the amplitude of any component should be equal across the head, but this is rarely true. The brain is a heterogenous organ, and, when functioning normally, expresses different components in different amounts. For example, especially with eyes closed, there is much more alpha posteriorly than anteriorly. This is a sign of normal, healthy functioning. Any significant deviation from this asymmetry is cause for consideration. As another example, there should be more beta frontally than posteriorly. Deviations from this, such as excess posterior beta, may be accompanied by different signs, such as possible anxiety or even depression. A third example of asymmetry is the left/right frontal asymmetry associated with positive mood.

Phase

Phase itself is an important metric. There are various methods of measuring phase. The traditional way to compute phase is to use the arctangent of the ratio of quadrature components derived from the FFT.

$$\text{Phase} = \text{Arc tan}\left(\frac{b}{a}\right)$$

The phase difference between two signals is simply:

$$\text{Phase\_difference} = \text{Arc tan}\left(\frac{b_2}{a_2}\right) - \text{Arc tan}\left(\frac{b_1}{a_1}\right)$$

Phase is a measure of the closeness of the peaks and valleys in two signals. Functionally, it reflects the speed of information sharing between the two sites.

Phase

- Various methods to compute.
- Attempts to extract phase relationship using mathematical technique.
- Stability and "wraparound" issues.
- FFT or quad digital filters.
- Reflects how well signals line up in time.
- Measure of speed of information sharing.
- Useful for synchrony training.

Sum of Channels

Adding two channels together in the time domain is a very efficient way to gain access to information regarding mutual activity. For example, if peaks and valleys line up, then the sum signal will be larger than either of the two initial signals. If the signals are uncorrelated, then this will not occur.

Sum of channels is an interesting contrast to the difference signal that is typically acquired using a bipolar connection. Figure 6.5 illustrates the data flow when the sum and difference of two channels are used for training.

Figure 6.7 shows the ratio of amplitudes of channel sum and difference for a range of phase values. This ratio is extremely sensitive to phase, and

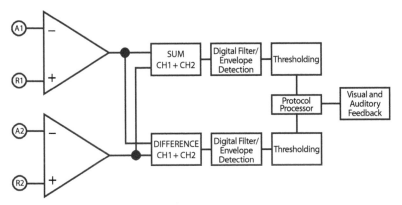

Figure 6.5 Method for computing sum and difference of two channels.

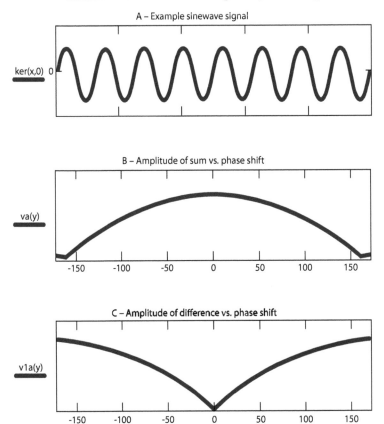

Figure 6.6 Effect of channel sum and difference on detecting phase relationship. Channel difference is maximally sensitive to phase shifts near zero.

Channel Difference

- Same as bipolar montage.
- Similar signals will cancel.
- Emphasizes differences.
- Useful for coherence downtraining.
- Cannot uptrain coherence with bipolar.
- Random (uncorrelated) signals: sum and difference signals will look the same.

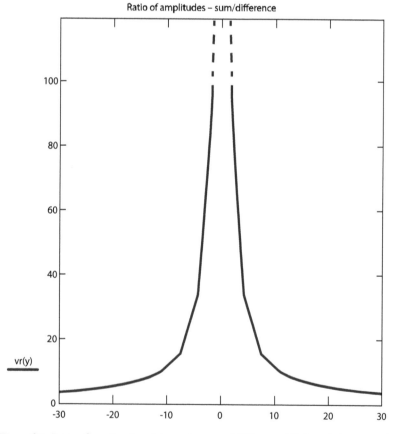

Figure 6.7 Ratio of amplitudes of channel sum and difference. Their ratio is extremely sensitive to phase near zero.

can detect when phases are exactly lined up (zero) by taking on an extremely large, theoretically unbounded, value.

Results with Two-Channel EEG and Sum/Difference Mode Using a Compressed Spectral Array

The compressed spectral array (CSA) is designed to provide a three-dimensional time/frequency representation of EEG signals, using a combination of frequency analysis, spline interpolation, and color-coded representation of signal amplitude. In a single display, typically one minute of EEG is displayed, with frequency as the horizontal axis, amplitude as the vertical axis, and time as the "z" axis. When a signal appears within a defined frequency band and has a "waxing" phase, then it appears as a color change on the display, with a three-dimensional representation of both its size and its time behavior. It is thus possible to see waxing and waning, and relationships between channels, in a visually clear format.

When sum/difference channel mode is used, the two signals viewed are transformed into their sum and difference signals, and displayed in the usual manner. When this is done, signals that are synchronous in both channels will emerge in the sum signal, and will tend to be small or invisible in the difference signal. In the BrainMaster, the signals can be viewed (and trained) in either the conventional two-channel mode, or in the sum/difference channel mode.

When playing back EEG data, it is possible to view it in either the conventional two-channel format or in the sum/difference format. This makes it possible to make playbacks in both modes and view the comparison. The visual differences between the two-channel BrainScapes and the sum/difference BrainScapes make it clearly evident when there is synchronous activity in any band. In the following examples, synchronous activity is evident in all bands. In addition to the expected alpha and related component bands, we are able to see synchronous high beta and gamma activity when it appears.

It can be shown that sum and difference signals are sensitive to both the amplitude and the phase of any signals that may be shared between the two sites. If signals are large and in phase, they will reinforce in the sum and be cancelled in the difference. The amplitude of the resulting sum and difference signals is thus an indicator of the degree of amplitude and phase similarity in the two channels. When the sum and difference signals are subjected to a frequency analysis, it is possible to separate the synchronous from the independent EEG activity in all frequency bands using the BrainScape display.

The following plots are derived from a playback of a BrainMaster MINI-Q session (eyes closed) with one-minute samples from each pair of sites.

They illustrate the use of sum/difference channel analysis and the BrainScape display in interpreting recordings from six pairs of sites: Fz/Cz, F3/F4, C3/C4, P3/P4, T3/T4, and O1/O2, with linked ear reference. In each pair, it is possible to discern which activity is dominant at each site, and which activity is common between the sites.

Color Plate 12 shows Fz and Cz in standard two-channel mode: the overall symmetry in the signal is evident, and rhythmic theta and alpha are visible. There is also a small amount of activity in the beta bands and a very small amount of gamma activity.

Color Plate 13 shows Fz and Cz in sum/difference channel mode: it is now clear the extent to which the energy is synchronous versus independent. For example, the right (difference) channel is almost entirely quiet above 30 Hz, yet the left (sum) channel is very active in this entire range. This indicates that this activity is almost entirely synchronous between Fz and Cz. Also, note the large synchronous burst at approximately 28 Hz.

Color Plate 14 shows F3 and F4 in standard two-channel mode: here, some asymmetry is evident, in that channel 2 (F4) is slightly larger overall than F3. Moderate theta activity and sporadic alpha bursts are evident. Tiny amounts of high beta and gamma activity are also visible.

Color Plate 15 shows F3 and F4 in sum/difference channel mode: synchronous theta and alpha are clear. The similarity between the right and left signals suggests the degree to which these frequencies are independent between these two leads. Note the single large synchronous burst of 40 Hz in the left signal that is clearly captured by this method.

Color Plate 16 shows C3 and C4 in standard two-channel mode: the appearance is largely symmetrical, with very little activity above 30 Hz.

Color Plate 17 shows C3 and C4 in sum/difference channel mode: synchronous theta, alpha, and SMR are evident. The small amount of gamma appears almost entirely synchronous, as it appears clearly on the left (sum) trace, yet is entirely missing from the right (difference) signal.

Color Plate 18 shows P3 and P4 in standard two-channel mode: the traces look largely similar. Note the small movement-related artifacts near the top of both traces, which produce a broad distribution of frequency noise.

Color Plate 19 shows P3 and P4 in sum/difference channel mode: the degree of synchrony at low frequencies is clearly evident. Note how the artifacts near the top of the displays are reinforced in the sum channel, yet are entirely missing from the right channel. This demonstrates the effectiveness of this technique in separating even very large common-mode signals from differential signals.

Color Plate 20 shows T3 and T4 in standard two-channel mode: the signals look largely alike, and include minimal activity above 30 Hz.

Color Plate 21 shows T3 and T4 in sum/difference channel mode: here, the independence of the signals is demonstrated by the appearance of strong alpha and up to 30 Hz in the right channel, which looks similar to the signals in the left channel. Similar appearance on the sum and difference is the hallmark of signals that are independent (uncorrelated).

Color Plate 22 shows O1 and O2 in standard two-channel mode: here, synchronous bursts of alpha are clearly evident in both channels.

Color Plate 23 shows O1 and O2 in sum/difference channel mode: the extreme degree of occipital alpha synchrony appears dramatically in the left versus right signals. A small amount of independent alpha does appear. Note how the artifact near the top saturates the left (sum) signal, yet is entirely gone in the right (difference) signal.

7

FOUNDATIONS OF
NEUROFEEDBACK PROTOCOLS

Neurofeedback has evolved as a clinical practice over almost 30 years, and certain protocols have become standard. Their effects and clinical utility are well known, and they have important roles, not just historically, but in current use. Most of these protocols are still in use, and many of them are in use in modified form. A review of these standard protocols provides a valuable overview of many of the principles of neurofeedback, as well as important historical perspective.

The protocol we call "alert" is known more generally as beta training. It consists of a reward on increasing beta, with inhibits placed on theta and high beta. This protocol is generally applied either in sites that show deficits of beta, or generally at C3 or Cz. It would not be used at C4, as this would pose the concern of overactivating the right hemisphere, possibly elevating mood issues such as negativity or irritability. This is one of the historical protocols used for ADD/ADHD dating from the mid 1980s. One of the possible issues with this protocol is the possibility of general overactivation of the client. If this protocol is used for an excessive period of time (depending on the site and the client's reactivity), then agitation may result. In such cases, this can be followed by the "focus" protocol, described below. It should also be noted that if beta training is conducted on the right hemisphere, there is a greater likelihood of overactivation because the right hemisphere tends to operate slightly slower than the left.

The "focus" protocol is essentially the same as "alert," except that the enhanced band is SMR rather than beta. This protocol can also be used at Cz or at C4. It is significant that beta training tends to be done at C3, while SMR training tends to be done at C4. The subjective experience of SMR training is somewhat "smoother" than beta training. The client tends to get a relaxed yet focused internal sense, which can be subjectively described as "cruising." This reflects the normal condition that the left hemisphere is somewhat faster than the right hemisphere. One of the possible issues with SMR training is that, if overdone, it can result in underactivation. If a client becomes drowsy or lethargic from SMR training, one option is to follow with a small amount of beta training.

It should also be noted that if SMR is trained on the left hemisphere, there may be a particularly underactivated response.

"Peak" is an interesting protocol that has been made possible by the availability of two-channel EEG systems. "Peak" consists of "alert" on the left channel and "focus" on the right. This approach therefore combines the benefits of "alert" and "focus," while avoiding some of the drawbacks. Generically referred to as "C3 beta C4 SMR," this protocol can generally be used with minimal risk, and for overall general benefits in both alertness and in focus.

"Relax" is the classical alpha protocol, supplemented with an inhibit on theta and an inhibit on high beta. It can be used anywhere, but is generally used posteriorly at the occipital or parietal leads. Alpha training should be done with caution in the frontal areas, due to the possibility of mood-related reactions and also because frontal alpha tends to be slower than in the back. This can be used anywhere that mid-range frequencies are to be reinforced, but its primarily value is in posterior alpha training for relaxation. It is generally used eyes-closed, but eyes-open alpha training, while not particularly common, is also used. This protocol is also useful when the primary goal is reduction of theta or high beta, as these are included in the protocol. For this reason, Walker (2011) used this protocol as part of a QEEG-based approach to migraines.

"Sharp" is a "squash" protocol that consists of inhibits placed on four bands, spanning the range from 4 to 20 Hz. Its primary purpose is as an activation protocol, taking advantage of the fact that lower-amplitude EEG signals tend to be at higher frequencies. Therefore, generally reinforcing reductions in EEG amplitude will tend to inhibit low frequencies, such as delta and theta, and possibly also alpha, if the threshold is set low enough. The lower the threshold, the more this protocol will tend to reinforce higher frequencies. Left frontal broadband downtraining, for example, can produce benefits in mood as one form of asymmetry training, as reported by Hammond and Baehr (2008).

Standard Protocols

- Alert C3—beta up; theta, high beta down.
- Deep Pz—(Penniston) alpha up, theta up.
- Focus C4—SMR up; theta, high beta down.
- Peak C3-C4—alpha coherence up.
- Peak2 C3-C4—alert and focus combined.
- Relax Oz—alpha up; theta, high beta down.
- Sharp Cz—broadband squash.

The "deep" protocol implements alpha/theta training of the type described by Penniston and others (Penniston and Kulkowski, 1989, 1990; Penniston et al., 1993; Scott and Kaiser, 1998; Scott et al., 2005). In particular, Scott and Kaiser (1998) found that the addition of a prior SMR enhancement protocol, such as the focus protocol described below, resulted in marked improvement with polysubstance abusers in an in-patient setting. This type of deep-states training is entirely different from the other "high-frequency" techniques just described. The purpose of the alpha/theta training is to allow the brain to experience moving beyond the alpha state, and to begin to produce predominantly theta. This is done over an extended time, typically more than ½ hour, and under supervision of a trained clinician. The clinician will introduce therapeutic suggestions, images, and visualizations before and after the induction of the deep state.

The theory behind this training is that while the brain is producing theta, the amygdala is in a relaxed state and cannot process negative emotions or fear. The neuronal dynamics are similar to those that take place when occipital alpha is produced by a reverberation between the lateral geniculate nucleus and the occipital cortex. However, in this case, the central brain location is subthalamic, so that by enhancing the theta rhythm, the brain is led to preoccupy the amygdale with a relaxation rhythm, with the attendant subjective changes. Among other changes associated with theta are loss of muscle tone and a hypnogogic state.

Thomas Edison was known to use a "theta biofeedback" technique for his own creative development. He would hold a brass ball in his hand, over a pie tin that was placed on the floor, and doze off in his easy chair. When he entered a hypnogogic state, and subsequently lost muscle tone, his hand would relax and release the ball, which would strike the plate and wake him. In this dreamlike state, he would then take a paper and pencil and write down his ideas. This was a source of some of his more unusual ideas, as this internalized, creative state led to unusual associations and concepts.

During an alpha/theta session, there is an event called "crossover" that is expected some time into the session. At this point, whereas the alpha is generally the largest rhythm, theta becomes the dominant rhythm. It appears that at this point, the alpha magnitude drops, leaving the theta as the largest component. It is when the client is in this crossed-over condition that the hypnogogic state occurs. When this transition from an alpha-dominant state to a theta-dominant state occurs, the practitioner should be attentive to the client, and monitor the client's progress and state changes. This aspect of client-practitioner interaction is unique to alpha-theta training, and is an important factor that distinguishes it from other forms of neurofeedback.

The following tables compare important factors that differ between low-frequency "deep-states" training and more conventional beta, SMR, or alpha training. Upon reviewing the differences, it is apparent that these are really two entirely different applications of neurofeedback. While conventional training is oriented toward achieving mental fitness and freedom from dysregulations, deep-states training is more of a personal exploration, directed toward internal change and the process of recovery. It should be kept in mind that neurofeedback is an art as well as a science, and that there is some latitude in how principles are applied when implementing clinical interventions.

Table 7.1 compares components, goals, and other basic attributes of the two training approaches. Deep-states training involves letting go and slowly entering an altered state. High-frequency training is an exercise that implies effort and achievement of a goal.

Table 7.2 compares the context, brain areas, and session characteristics. Deep-states training involves continued total immersion and a trancelike state. High-frequency training consists typically of trials and can have a game-like quality.

Table 7.3 compares aspects such as volition, eye condition, and the end state of the training session.

"Squash" Protocols

The "squash" protocol is a family of designs that take advantage primarily of changes that occur when an EEG rhythm is reduced in amplitude. It was originally described by Maust (1999), and has been incorporated into many other designs since then. Among the more interesting recent related developments has been the multiple inhibit, which is described below.

The concept behind this protocol is that there is no specific "enhance" band defined at all. What are defined are bands that are downtrained, in

Table 7.1 Basic attributes of low-frequency versus high-frequency training

Characteristics	Low-frequency training	High-frequency training
Components	Alpha: reinforce Theta: reinforce	Beta: reinforced SMR: reinforced Theta: inhibited
Goal	Deeper awareness	Balance, control, alertness
Level of effort	Effortless, letting go	Effort, relaxed
Speed of response	Brain responds slowly, feedback can be slow	Brain responds quickly, rapid feedback
Use of feedback	Primarily an indicator	Want to "crank" thresholds and perform
Reward	Generally 80 %	Generally 50–60 %
Type of feedback	Mostly "yes," some "no"	Mostly "no," some "yes"

Table 7.2 Context, application, and other characteristics of low-frequency versus high-frequency training

Characteristics	Low-frequency training	High-frequency training
Trainee context	Immersion into relaxed state	Tuning, improving brain
Application	Exploration and recovery	Mental fitness
Brain areas	Parietal, occipital	Motor area
Modality	Auditory, trancelike	Visual, game-like
Sessions	30 minutes to 3 hours, no breaks	20–30 minutes, may have breaks
Relaxation	Total relaxation	Relaxation with muscle tone
Environment	Quiet, low lighting	Normal surrounding
Clinical use	Deep-seated issues, recovery	Attention, depression, other

Table 7.3 Volitional and related elements of low-frequency versus high-frequency training

Characteristics	Low-frequency training	High-frequency training
Volition	Abandon volition	Has volitional element
Self-improvement	Awareness, oneness, growth	Peak performance
Eyes	Eyes closed	Eyes open
Crossovers	Yes (from alpha state to theta state)	No
Increase	Look for 2× to 3×	Optional sustained increase
End state	Altered state of consciousness	Awake and alert state
Spatial	Widespread in space (brain)	Localized in space (brain)
Follow-on goal	Experience altered state now, reap follow-on benefits	Ability to reproduce state during daily life
Age	Not done with children	All ages

that the reward is produced when the band energy is below some value. Coming from the old model of "train one component up, keep the others down," this approach may not make sense. However, from an overall view of the concentration/relaxation cycle, it is perfectly reasonable. It is based on the understanding that when EEG amplitudes are reduced, it reflects activation, and also desynchronization of the underlying neuronal populations. There is also a tendency to produce higher frequencies because of the relationship between frequency and amplitude that we see in the EEG.

When doing squash training, there is a model that is similar to that of a "bench press." The client puts (moderate) effort into making the signal go down, and, when it does, a point and/or sound is rewarded. Then, the client can relax briefly. Thus, this tends to be a "trials" oriented approach. This approach is generally oriented toward improved mental fitness and acuity and positive mood. Depending on the site of the sensor, that region of the brain will tend to be activated. For example, doing a squash on the left frontal area, such as F3 or F7, would be expected to lead to a positive mood by activating the left dorsolateral frontal areas responsible for approach behavior and positive tone.

Multiple Inhibit Protocols

Multiple inhibits are widely used, and consist of a protocol in which many bands are set as inhibits. In a system with eight programmable bands, it would not be uncommon to set seven of them as inhibits, and have a single reward band. When using multiple inhibits, the contingency percentage is generally set low, such as for a 10 percent rate of inhibition. Therefore, these bands are not really being used to "downtrain" those frequencies. Rather, they are being used to keep the brain within a stable range of function. When using multiple inhibits, it is common to change the reward band and to use an empirical approach to determine the subjective effects on the client. This approach has resulted in some unusual protocols, including the "ILF" protocol described later.

Use of Overlapping Bands

In some protocol designs, the bands may overlap. This may even include an enhance band that overlaps with one or more inhibit bands. To a simple view that requires enhance bands and inhibit bands to be distinct, this may cause some confusion. For example, it is possible to enhance a band such as 7–13 Hz, while inhibiting theta from 4–8, and low beta from 12–15. It is even possible to both reinforce and inhibit the same band. While this might be perceived as creating a conflict or cancelling out training effects, this is not the case. Because different bands can have different thresholds, it is possible to meet all training conditions, even when bands overlap. Generally, in such cases, the thresholds for the inhibit bands will be larger than those for the reinforcement, so that the training message becomes "make more of this, but not too much."

Multiple Thresholds

Multiple thresholds can be used to create more complex and informative feedback, providing an element of proportional feedback. This allows the trainee to receive information related to "how much" or "how well" the training is proceeding. For example, in an inhibit protocol, it is possible to set thresholds at successively lower levels, and to introduce additional sounds with each level. As the trainee reduces the component, the sounds can become more complex, for example producing a "chord" of notes rather than a single note. Tom Brownback has developed a family of protocols that includes over 100 distinct designs, each tailored to a particular way of shaping the frequency content of the EEG (Brownback, 2010).

Infra-Low and Infra-Slow (ILF/ISF) Training

ILF/ISF training is an approach that was first developed empirically, and has gained clinical acceptance since its introduction by the Othmers (Othmer and Othmer, 2008; Smith, 2011). ILF/ISF training is controversial for several reasons. One is that there is dispute regarding the validity of recording signals in the very low ranges (0.001 Hz) and attributing them to valid brain sources. A second issue is that its clinical application tends to be guided by experience, not by rote procedure. With regard to the low signal frequency ranges, it has been noted previously that very slow potentials are generally not regarded as "rhythmic," but can be looked upon as shifts or fluctuations rather than oscillations. The use of the time constant in these protocols is primarily used to remove higher frequencies and to isolate the occasional shifts in potential from more rapid fluctuations. Therefore, the time constant is more relevant than the corner frequency. Thus, a frequency corner of, for example, 0.05 Hz does not mean that the signal is oscillating repeatedly at cycle of 20 seconds, but rather that a time constant on the order of 20 seconds is being used to ensure that shifts that are detected and reinforced are significant fluctuations, not small changes.

Synchrony Training

Synchrony training requires at least two channels of EEG to be monitored, processed, and used for feedback. It is not possible to do synchrony training with one channel. In particular, it is not possible to train synchrony using a "bipolar" hookup, such as T3 active and T4 reference. A bipolar connection can only downtrain synchrony, and can never uptrain synchrony. Thus, at least two channels are required, and each channel is typically recorded in a "monopolar" fashion, with a neutral reference such as an ear or linked ears. Synchrony training can also be done with more than two channels. The BrainMaster Atlantis 4×4 can be used to acquire and train four channels of synchrony. Also, the Open Focus Synchrony Trainer can be used to acquire five channels of EEG and combine them in hardware, providing one virtual EEG channel of output for training. This is described in more detail below.

Generally, synchrony training is done involving both hemispheres (left and right) of the brain. Typical active lead locations for two-channel training are, for example, C3 and C4. This would train primarily the motor strip. However, other choices include P3 and P4 (primarily the parietal areas), or O1 and O2 (primarily the occipital areas). When four channels are used, training can be both inter-hemispheric (between the hemispheres) and intra-hemispheric (within a hemisphere). An example of a four-channel inter- and intra-hemispheric connection would be F3, F4, P3, and P4.

Any frequency component band or bands can be trained using synchrony training. The most common frequency band is alpha (8–12 Hz), since it is known that alpha synchrony is accompanied by relaxation, mental clarity, and similar benefits. Training synchronous theta (4–7 Hz) and delta (1–4 Hz) is not recommended, as these components are often associated with drowsiness, distraction, and are often seen in cases of attention deficit and cognitive disorders. Beta (15–30 Hz) is also not commonly trained for synchrony because beta waves are more localized in general and diffuse beta is associated with such things as anxiety and tension. Gamma (35–45 Hz) can be trained for synchrony, and gamma synchrony is associated with mental clarity, problem-solving, and higher cognitive function. Synchrony training of alpha and gamma together is an emerging technique, which can combine the beneficial effects of each approach, enhancing both relaxation and mental clarity. These components can be easily trained by using the two bands as enhance ("go") components in a synchrony protocol.

Synchrony can be trained by using various built-in metrics such as coherence, similarity, spectral correlation, and comodulation. The simplest method, however, is to do synchrony training using channel recombination (adding and subtracting raw EEG waveforms) as a simple and easy to learn technique.

One-Person Synchrony Training

One person can do synchrony training with two or more channels. The simplest method is to acquire two channels of EEG. It is customary to acquire each channel in a "monopolar" fashion and to set up an appropriate protocol for synchrony training.

One-Person Two-Channel Synchrony Training

One person can do basic synchrony training with two channels by using two monopolar hookups as shown. The exact active leads can be C3 and C4, P3 and P4, or O1 and O2, for example. In this application, frontal leads (e.g. F3 and F4) are not common and are not recommended.

Once the sensors are placed as shown, several protocols can be used to uptrain synchrony. One of them is the built-in protocol called "peak," which

139

Basic 2-channel connection:

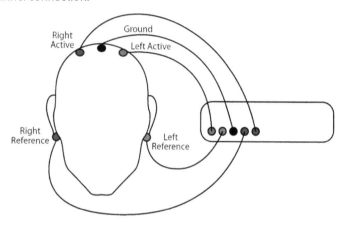

Figure 7.1 Basic two-channel connections for one person.

trains using a "metric" such as coherence or similarity. The user can start with this protocol and then choose any of the available metrics, such as "pure coherence," "training/similarity," "spectral correlation coefficient (SCC), or "comodulation." Any of these will train the EEG of the two channels to have similar characteristics, as follows:

- Pure coherence—will train for stability of the phase separation between the two channels.
- Training coherence—will train for zero phase separation and similar amplitude.
- Spectral correlation—will train for similar spectral energy.
- Comodulation—will train for similar amplitude variations between the two channels.
- Phase—when trained down, will train the signals to be in phase.

The "peak" protocol provides sound feedback, indicating that the signals are increasingly similar. The coherence threshold should be adjusted for optimal feedback. It is not possible to use "autothresholding" with coherence, as this is not advisable for clinical reasons. Rather, it is best to set the threshold continually to find the best level for training.

Use of Sum Channel Mode

The approach that will be emphasized here is to use the "sum channel" mode. This mode is chosen by simply setting sum channel mode "ON" in the data channels control panel. When two channels are used, the choice of sum channel mode to "ON" is all that is required to enter this mode of operation.

When this option used, set up the protocol as follows:

• Data channels—two channels of EEG.
• Sum channel mode "ON."
• Training protocol—channel 1 "go" on the component of interest.
• Training protocol—channel 2 "stop" on the component of interest.

When sum channel mode is turned on, the EEG channels are recomputed so that channel 1 becomes the sum and channel 2 becomes the difference. In other words:

• 1 + 2 becomes channel 1.
• 1 – 2 becomes channel 2.

When the channels are "recombined" in this manner, the displays and computations proceed as normal, except that the waveforms used are the algebraic ("arithmetic") sum and difference signals. This method will up-train the sum of the channels and downtrain the difference. This will reward when the two channels are synchronized, and will tend to train them to be the same in frequency and phase, as well as being maximum amplitude. An example of the training screen is shown below. Note that the waveforms are labeled as the SUM and DIFF respectively, and that channel 1 is being trained up ("+" in the left thermometer) and channel 2 is being trained down ("–" in the right thermometer). See Color Plate 24

One-Person Four-Channel Synchrony Training

One person can do advanced synchrony training with four channels as shown.

Note that this connection uses linked ears as a convenience. The "jumper" wire is used to combine the ear references into a single "linked-ears" reference that is used for each of the four channels. The four active channels used in this example are F3, F4, P3, and P4. Other choices could be used, for example C3, C4, Fz, and Pz.

When sum channel mode is used with four channels, there are two possibilities, called "split" and "combine."

In "split" mode, the channels are mapped as follows:

• 1 + 2 becomes channel 1.
• 1 – 2 becomes channel 2.
• 3 + 4 becomes channel 3.
• 3 – 4 becomes channel 4.

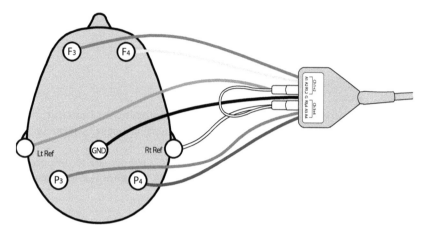

Figure 7.2 Basic connections for four-channel training.

With this mode, one would typically uptrain channels 1 and 3 and downtrain channels 2 and 4.

In "combine" mode, the channels are mapped as follows:

- 1 + 2 + 3 + 4 becomes channel 1.
- 1 − 2 becomes channel 2.
- (1 + 2) − (3 + 4) becomes channel 3.
- 3 − 4 becomes channel 4.

In this mode, one would typically uptrain channel 1 and downtrain channels 2, 3, and 4.

Two Persons

There are various ways to train two people with synchrony training. The goals are twofold. The first is that each individual is doing synchrony training within his or her own brain. The second is that the two individuals are doing synchrony training between each other. The simplest method, to use two channels for two people, satisfies the second goal, but not the first.

Two-Person Two-Channel Synchrony Training

It is possible to do synchrony training between two people with a two-channel EEG. In this case, each individual is not getting synchrony training within themselves. However, they are training synchrony with each other. A possible connection is as shown. Note that a jumper would be used so that each of the grounds is going into the same connection. As an alternative, the two individuals could be connected with a separate lead. Or, they could hold hands or touch in some other way to be at the same ground potential.

When two people are connected in this way, any of the preceding two-channel synchrony protocols can be used to train the two EEG signals into synchrony. The following is an actual screen of a two-person training session using this type of connection. The protocol used was the standard "peak" protocol. Observe that the two EEG waveforms look different in frequency content. The partner on the left has more alpha waves, and the partner on the right has more SMR energy. Note that the BrainMirror shows this difference. By using the "peak" protocol, the trainees get a reward sound when the coherence between their EEG's is large. This encourages them to have a consistent phase relationship between their EEG waves. An alternative scheme could be to use the "comodulation," which would encourage their EEG energy to wax and wane together. Comodulation is an easier condition to meet, since it does not require that the waves are phase-locked, only that they rise and fall at the same time.

See Color Plate 25 for an example screen of two people doing synchrony training, with a total of two channels.

Two-Person Four-Channel Synchrony Training

It is also possible to train two people with synchrony training with four channels, in which each person is doing synchrony training within themselves, and also with each other. In this use, you could use either the "split" or the "combine" sum channel mode. If you use "split," you would uptrain the two sum channels (channels 1 and 3) and downtrain the two difference channels (channels 2 and 4). This emphasizes the individual synchrony, not the combined synchrony.

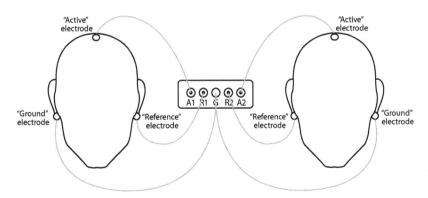

Figure 7.3 Connections for two-person training, using one channel per individual.

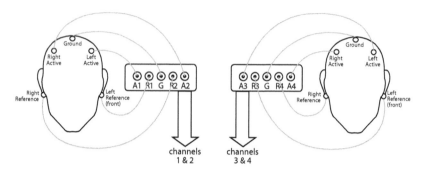

Figure 7.4 Two-person training with two channels per individual, for a total of four channels.

To use the "combine" method, one would uptrain channel 1 and downtrain the other three channels. This would train the couple to maximize their synchrony together, and also to maximize their individual synchrony.

Application Focus—Neurofeedback Applications for Optimal Performance

This section describes some basic considerations and operational details for the use of neurofeedback in relation to performance improvement or mental fitness. This will help the reader to gain a perspective on non-medical, non-therapeutic uses of neurofeedback. Generally, neurofeedback will be used in order to acquaint trainees with desirable mental states, and to help them to learn to achieve and recognize these states. Our approach to training these states is based upon the concepts of flexibility and appropriateness, and does not appeal to the notion of good versus bad brainwaves. No particular brain state is good or bad, in its own context. What matters is being able to achieve an appropriate state at the appropriate time. There is an element of creating beneficial habits that become second nature, so that desirable brain states occur at the appropriate times without overt effort. A recent study illustrating the value of this approach was reported by Cochran (2012). The benefits of SMR training, as well as theta reduction and high beta reduction, for example, were described and applied in a setting that provided significant positive results for a group of executives. The participants reported improved focus, productivity, and sleep, as well as reductions in impulsivity and anxiety.

This section is intended to provide information for the neurotherapist or coach, as well as the trainee. It does not provide details on how to organize a training program, or exactly how or when to administer neurofeedback treatments. Rather, it provides a brief description of the basic protocols and techniques, with a short explanation of the manner of use and the anticipated benefits. The neurotherapist and trainee should be able to work together to provide a simple sequence of trainings, progressing from simple to more complex, and to suit the needs at hand. At a minimum, trainees will likely do simple SMR or alpha training, and a basic type of "squash" protocol to learn mental activation. There is sufficient flexibility and expandability in the available neurofeedback systems to accommodate a growing and advancing personal plan that can easily extend to many months, and years, as training progresses and the trainee learns more depth and sophistication.

What are the mental tasks associated with optimal performance? There are many. There is the need to take in the overall layout of mental tasks and to execute subtasks when needed. Similar mental processes underlie various tasks, such as firing an arrow, hitting a golf shot, or playing basketball. When making a golf putt, for example, there is the need to calibrate oneself to each hole, and to relate the distance and direction to one's personal position at the outset. Then, there is the need to stand before the ball and be still, and prepare for a brief moment of highly precise action. But this action must be undertaken in a relaxed, automatic fashion, free of the encumbrances of overt thought. The mind cannot consciously process a golf stroke as it happens; it must be automatic, practiced, and sure. Finally, after each shot, the individual must again relax, process the activity, and prepare for the next. The golfer must be able to carry out repeated, precise, difficult maneuvers without tiring or becoming frustrated or angry. The successful and satisfying completion of this complex series of tasks is facilitated by being able to achieve the relevant brain state at the relevant time, and being able to move gracefully and freely from state to state. In terms of the coin and funnel analogy described in Chapter 2, the individual primes each funnel, sets up the coins, and then releases them, so that the task execution is essentially one of falling into action as a release of potential energy that produces action. This is at the core of golf, or of any sport or activity that relies on precise automatic action.

As a result, what we describe here are basic techniques and tools, for personal fitness, awareness, and improvement. In the context of golf, this becomes neurofeedback for peak performance. But what we are really teaching here is neurofeedback for better living. Golf is simply a phase of life that presents its own unique challenges, measures, and rewards. But in the sense that, as an activity, it asks us to be relaxed, focused, directed, composed, and efficient, it is merely a special case of regular life, and nothing more. In other words, get better at mental fitness and you become better at golf. Become better at golf and you might become better at life.

Rather than providing a prescription or plan for personal improvement, this section presents a survey of techniques, their characteristics, and their possible use. From this collection, the trainer and trainee can pick and choose those that seem most appropriate, and incorporate them into the program. It is expected that training plans will evolve and grow along with the experiences of the trainers and trainees who use them, and that continued progress will lead to a variety of approaches and plans designed to suit individuals and groups at all stages along the various roads to personal progress and improvement.

Basic Considerations

It is important to understand that the brain is a dynamic entity, much like the body, and that it has a variety of tasks and ways to achieve them. It needs to be able to shift quickly and effectively between particular states in the pursuit of task performance, satisfaction, health, and sustainability. So we will not try to identify certain frequencies as "good" and others as "bad," or try to eliminate some and enhance others for this type of reasoning. We will look to train the flexibility to enter and leave identifiable brain states at appropriate times, and to be able to recognize when this happens. We would not, for example, train a basketball player to run around the court with an arm in the air at all times, just because the basket is up there. We must train the player to have the arm in the appropriate place at the appropriate time, and to be ready to move it there quickly. We need to train flexibility and appropriateness, not a fixed set of brain frequencies.

Previous work (Chartier et al., 1997) has identified effective neurofeedback training of elite golfers, as well as helping them to achieve what is called an "iceberg profile" on the profile of mood states (POMS). In this report, 14 out of 15 participants reported significant improvement in their game as measured by pre- and post-training scores. Improvements were also reported in the Symptom Checklist 90, particularly in the obsessive-compulsive scale. This demonstrated the value of neurofeedback training in a peak performance context, when used in a golfing situation.

What follows is a series of brief descriptions of specific protocols and methods, with an indication of how these could be applied as part of a comprehensive performance improvement plan. This may be viewed as a shopping list, or a starting point for the discussion and planning of specific programs for golf improvement. It is hoped that trainers and administrators will be able to extract from these descriptions sufficient information to create the basic plan for training, and to begin to explore neurofeedback training and its benefits as part of a comprehensive plan of performance improvement.

Note that all neurofeedback training is, at its heart, relaxation training. Whatever the location and the frequencies trained, there is an element of relaxation, in that cortical brain cells produce measurable voltages only when they act in unison. In order to act in synchrony, they must relax inhibition, allowing post-synaptic potentials to be expressed in response to

146

thalamo-cortical reverberation. By allowing the brain to relax and produce endogenous rhythms in various combinations, it is possible to train specific changes in brain state in particular locations, and in particular ways. But what is always happening is that the brain is finding its own way. Neurofeedback never forces anything to happen. It shows the brain when the desired state is present. Training mostly consists of relaxing, letting go, and allowing the equipment and the brain to work together. In this way, there is a naturalness to the learning, and what is thus learned is generally retained. Having learned to relax and achieve particular states, the trainee is thus prepared to undertake a task with a sense of confidence, automaticity, and simplicity. It is truly learning, in the best meaning of the term.

One of the lessons of golf, as well as life, is that it is not supposed to be hard. We learn to think and act smarter, not harder. Neurofeedback complements this concept by providing additional mental and brain tools, allowing the player to proceed in a more natural, effortless manner, toward performance that has fewer errors, fewer distractions, and more productivity.

Alpha Relaxation

This is the basic relaxing, one-channel or two-channel alpha feedback (8–12 Hz) using relaxing feedback sounds with real-time amplitude feedback. Eyes are generally closed. This will be done with theta inhibition, using the standard relax protocol. The trainee closes eyes, relaxes, and allows the tones to come. Voices may be flutes, cello, viola, seashore, "spacey" sounds, etc. This will achieve a state of general relaxation, while avoiding reinforcement of the lower-frequency theta activity associated with deeper, inner connectedness, or distractibility. Generally, O1/O2, P3/P4, or C3/C4 will be used with two- or three-minute segments, optionally separated by pauses.

Alpha training allows trainees to learn to relax in general and achieve a state that is generally healthy. For example, when walking the course, when planning shots, when working with scoring, it is generally a good thing to be relaxed yet alert. Achieving and maintaining this state is helpful for generally reducing stress and its associated effects, and will also help to minimize the effects of anxieties, anger, disappointment, or other negative emotions that may arise.

Alpha Coherence

This is a more specific type of alpha training, achieving a coherent state between the left and right hemispheres, in the alpha (8–12 Hz) band. Eyes are again generally closed, and "peak" protocol is used. Generally, O1/O2, P3/P4, or C3/C4 can be used. Trainees typically uptrain coherence in one- or two-minute segments, optionally separated by pauses.

This coherent alpha state is a state of well-poised readiness, as well as relaxation. It is associated with improved creativity, sense of well-being, and the ability to perform effectively. It has been seen in Zen monks and similar meditative and contemplative individuals, and seen in conjunction with various forms of meditation. However, the alpha state is not equivalent to meditation. It is a particular state, and meditators may or may not achieve particularly high levels of alpha coherence, depending on the style of meditation.

This type of training can also be used in a general situation in which it is desirable to reduce the high beta and theta, as primary goals. Walker (2011) reported on a series of patients with migraines who exhibited excess high beta at particular sites. As a strategy to reduce this, he applied the general alpha protocol at the affected sites, which resulted in the effective reduction of beta. As will be discussed in Chapter 11, by varying thresholds, it is possible to adjust the amount of sensitivity of the feedback to particular components, effectively "titrating" neurofeedback to suit the needs at hand.

Alpha as Placebo

In the 1980s, a study was published that claimed to have demonstrated that alpha biofeedback was basically a placebo effect. Plotkin and Rice (1981) were able to show significant reductions in trait and state anxiety, and that these changes were highly correlated with trainees' ratings of perceived success at the feedback task. At the same time, these positive results were uncorrelated to the direction or magnitude of the changes in alpha activity. This showed that when trainees were able to gain effective awareness and control of their alpha rhythm, benefits in reduced anxiety could be expected. While the authors interpreted this as supporting a placebo interpretation, this is not at all clear when the model of flexibility and appropriateness is applied. Neurofeedback is not a simple matter of making "big things small" or "small things big." It is a process by which the brain learns self-regulation and begins to instrument new capabilities based upon this awareness. The direction is less critical than the acquisition of the task. To interpret this experiment as placebo is similar to having one group do pushups and another do pullups. While both groups would report benefits of exercise, it would not follow that "pushing or pulling on things has a placebo effect."

Focus—14 Hz ("SMR")

The basic focus protocol, such as used by Cochran (2012), provides enhancement training of the 12–15 low beta range with eyes open, using a single channel placed at C4 or, optionally, Cz. This protocol also inhibits theta and high beta. It is possible to emphasize the inhibits by adjusting the low beta theshold to zero, which is equivalent to setting the target percent time over threshold for low beta to 100 percent, effectively removing it from the feedback contingency. As the low beta threshold is increased, the element of focus and concentration is increased. This type of training is generally done using a simple sound, such as a click or beep, as the primary feedback. A preferred coaching strategy with focus training is to have the client relax and "allow the sounds to come." Each point earned thus produces an incremental learning experience. A typical reward rate is to achieve 600 to 800 points in a 20-minute session.

Overall, this is a good "relaxed, focused concentration" protocol. It is used extensively (Lubar et al., 1995; Sterman, 2000) in work with those with difficulty paying attention, and those who are hyperactive. Arns et al. (2012) also reported on the use of an SMR protocol when other, more directed protocols are not indicated. Specifically, the centrally generated SMR (sensorimotor rhythm) has been shown to be associated with the brain's "intent to remain still." It can be trained in cats and other mammals, and is a basic relaxation rhythm of the motor system. For example, it is extinguished when a contralateral limb is moved, shaking, etc. Training this rhythm teaches a deep relaxation of the sensorimotor system, and thus involves stillness of the body. This typically leaves the trainee in a relaxed and still, yet focused, alert, and ready state. This is one example of a state that may be regarded as "the zone." When the trainee is able to achieve and sustain good performance in this task, he or she may experience a sense of "cruising" or "getting into it," which is automatic, yet responds to the direction of the trainee's will to find and hold it.

Associated as it is with stillness, plus having theta reduction, this training protocol is often associated with training to help people function in a structured, academic, or attention-demanding environment. For example, it is commonly used with schoolchildren, businesspeople, etc. In a sports application, it helps to achieve a still, focused state for appropriate times. For example, in any seminar or workshop setting, when discussing concepts, or when studying specific shots, planning, and reasoning, this state of relaxed yet alert, focused concentration enhances the ability to think, reason, and reach good conclusions.

Excess SMR?

A participant in a workshop was being evaluated using EEG, and exhibited the deviation of having "excess SMR." The individual had a resting, eyes-open SMR that was on the order of 1.5 standard deviations high, compared to the general population. When questioned, the participant identified himself as a pediatric psychiatrist, who had developed and refined the skill of attentive listening to clients, regardless of how long they spoke or what they were saying. This trait of having out-of-the-ordinary attention skills was revealed in his resting EEG. When we attempted to reinforce a reduction in SMR to bring the EEG more toward "normal," this individual reported a sense of becoming more agitated and uncomfortable. This reflected a difference of personal style, and suggested that this person's brain knew where it was comfortable, even if it was not operating at the "normal" level with regard to this rhythm. This highlights the importance of individual considerations, both in interpreting QEEG and also in planning and administering neurofeedback. There is no "one-size-fits-all" approach to neurofeedback, even in the simplest of circumstances.

Low-Frequency Inhibition ("Squash")

This simple approach focuses on learning the task of reducing the low frequency EEG in the theta (4–7 Hz) band as the primary task. Eyes are generally open. Trainees learn to experience the feel of moments of low theta, observing a bar graph and hearing a sound when this is sustained. This can be implemented with any protocol that includes theta inhibition, such as the alert, focus, or relax protocols by setting the reinforcement threshold very low. Reducing theta is associated with decreased distractibility and the ability to focus on one thing at a time.

At any time that a trainee is faced with the need to limit concentration to a single item, this training is helpful. It is associated with a decrease in distractibility, less tendency for the mind to run in all directions, and improvement in the ability to have a single thing in mind without switching around. It is also associated with stillness and rest, because the theta wave also serves to detect eye movements, head movements, and other types of activity. Thus, theta inhibition encourages the head, neck, eyes, etc. to be still and quiet, while the brain also settles down and stops shifting around.

This protocol is generally used with simple tone or discrete sounds (clicks, etc.) and is generally done eyes open. The trainee should try to experience the "body feel" of when the theta is reduced. It is an indescribable yet pleasant and still feeling. It may be associated with focusing of thought and a sense of distractions fading away. It may be thought of as a "pushup" for the brain (actually a push-down), and should be practiced for a minute or two, with brief pauses if desired.

Broadband "Squash"

This extends the low-frequency squash technique to a broader band (4–20 Hz). This can be done with the sharp protocol. This helps trainees to achieve a state of overall EEG quietude, which is physiologically associated with a neuronal state of readiness, acuity of response, and being poised for action. The placement can be anywhere on the head, but is often used centrally or frontally. Skilled archers and pilots, for example, have been shown to have a state of overall EEG quieting (and a shift to beta frequencies) during the moments before well-executed skilled actions. This training emphasizes entering that state of optimal readiness for a difficult task, such as a golf swing, and learning to maintain that state in preparation for the execution of skilled actions.

This is best viewed as a special task, to be done for a brief (30-second or one-minute) trial, followed by a pause. It is a form of "bench pressing" for the mind. During the pause, the brain may produce alpha, and this is, in fact, beneficial. The brain will learn to focus and squash when asked, then to relax and produce alpha (a form of "post-reward synchronization") in the relaxation phase. The important point is to learn the concentration/relaxation cycle, not to achieve a permanent state of low EEG.

Individuals who have learned to achieve the concentration/relaxation cycle in an automatic and habitual manner may demonstrate the ability to execute difficult tasks faster, with better repeatability and with more stamina (Sterman et al., 1994).

Alpha/Theta Training

As has been described previously, alpha/theta training does not fit into the "mold" of more general alpha, beta, or SMR reinforcement protocols. This approach will usually be done in particular situations, under specific supervision of a clinician managing the trainee. Using a one-channel protocol ("deep"), both alpha and theta are reinforced, leading to an altered state of consciousness. Eyes are always closed, and sessions extend for longer times (30 or more minutes). Feedback sounds are deep, soothing instruments using selected or specially designed sounds to enhance the ethereal aspect of the experience. This type of training should be done in conjunction with psychotherapeutic, experiential, or related work. The focus of this work involves access to deeper, inner states, subsequent processing, and changes in awareness, etc. Unlike typical high-frequency training, this approach should be used by a specially trained clinician who is experienced in handling the personal changes and internal experiences that the feedback can elicit.

Alpha/theta training will be used in cases where a trainee desires to pursue specific issues, which may center around internal thoughts, feelings, memories, or other issues. This experience continues the basic relaxation achieved in alpha training, and further allows the brain to slow down in frequency and to produce diffuse theta waves. Normally associated with distractability, daydreaming, and creativity, when theta waves are trained for a continued period, the trainee achieves internal connectedness that may also be associated with feelings of dreamlike states, imagery, free association, and intuitive thoughts. Alpha/theta training is generally followed by a period of reactivation, discussion, experiential work, or other processes that incorporate the new information into the trainee's continued processing, allowing the benefits of the new awareness to be achieved. Possible abreaction may include a sense of disconnectedness, anxiety, or similar negative affect. Drowsiness may persist after the training if sufficient reactivation is not achieved afterward.

Photic, Auditory, and Magnetic Stimulation

Photic, auditory, or even electromagnetic stimulation can be used as an addition to neurofeedback training. These may elicit a frequency-following or "entrainment" effect on the EEG, although such effects may be temporary. These are useful to acquaint the brain with particular types of states, and to provide what is essentially a brain "massage," which may be stimulating or relaxing. Stimulation may also produce a general inhibitory effect, and may result in a reduction of low frequencies. However, after some time, effects may tend to go away if no learning mechanism, such as operant conditioning, is instrumented. For more effective stimulus-assisted neurofeedback training and for more lasting learning, EEG-controlled systems can be considered.

Photic Stimulation

The photic stimulator is capable of delivering controlled photic stimulation under EEG control. In the use for theta reduction, the glasses can be programmed to flash at an appropriate rate (typically 12–15 Hz) when the theta activity exceeds threshold. This has an automatic effect of reducing theta in the trainee, and helping him or her to learn to enter and recognize the state of reduced theta. It is an assist that helps the trainee to enter the state, by a "non-volitional" method, hence independent of the trainee's effort or volition (see Chapter 13). After a short period of such training, one of the conventional neurofeedback protocols can be used to reinforce the learning and allow the training to progress from the assisted state into further learned states. Patrick (1996), for example, reported benefits using photic stimulation with ADHD clients.

This approach provides special clues for enhancing or inhibiting rhythms, and adds a direct manipulation of the EEG, in what is closer to "classical conditioning" than "operant conditioning." Thus, as a very basic reward or inhibit mechanism, the brain can be coaxed into particular states without the trainee's conscious effort, providing a rapid and efficient way to either start training ("training wheels"), or to accelerate the progress of training ("personal coach").

"Interactor" Vibrotactile Cushion

This auxiliary feedback device will operate with all of the above protocols and techniques. It provides a kinesthetic feedback delivered with a strong vibrotactile stimulator. Feedback is felt, not seen or heard, and can be delivered to the hand, arm, leg, back, or any other suitable body surface. It provides feedback that is pleasant and easy to sense, and also does not depend on the brain's auditory or visual processing system in order to process the information. In other words, it provides direct body feedback so that the body participates more fully in the feedback learning process.

It is notable that this type of feedback provides the opportunity for the trainee to work with eyes closed, and in an essentially silent environment. The mind is truly stilled, and the visual and auditory senses are not active. This provides a very peaceful, focused type of training, and allows the trainee to focus on inner awareness, without the distractions of having to view, listen to, or process some sensory input. This is a direct "brain-to-body" link, and has qualities and benefits all its own.

We also look at this type of feedback as a "pat on the back." The trainee obtains a rapid, pleasant, and reinforcing feedback that directly appeals the physical sense of having done the right thing. Very little (or no) instruction is necessary, as everyone knows the inner reward sense that is achieved with reassuring and well-deserved tactile feedback, especially when it is so closely coupled to the task being reinforced. Depending on the protocol and type of feedback used, the trainee may given a "pat," whether they focus and reduce theta, achieve a state of bodily stillness and relaxation, succeed in achieving a state of coherence, or whatever the protocol is doing. There is also a natural continuity with physical guidance, coaching, and reinforcement that may be given by the coach himself or herself, in which the body is an essential element in the learning.

153

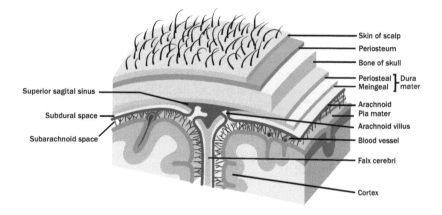

Plate 1 Anatomic view of brain and overlying skull and scalp.

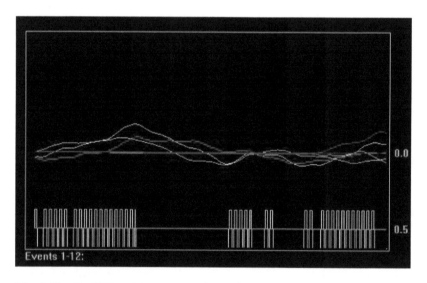

Plate 2 Detail of SCP training screen and reward method. SCP signals for F3, F4, P3, and P4 are shown in blue, yellow, green, and red respectively. Total SCP signal is in white. Rewards are earned when the total SCP potential is rising (bottom indicator).

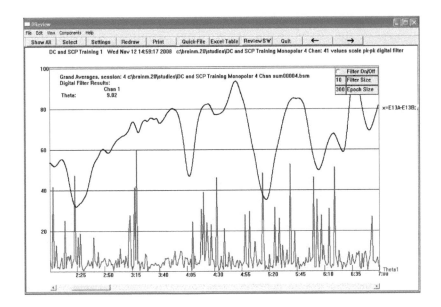

Plate 3 Simultaneous slow cortical potential (SCP) (black) and filtered magnitude of theta wave (blue) for a five-minute training epoch. Note that the SCP signals exhibit a characteristically different type of response when compared to conventional magnitude-based training variables.

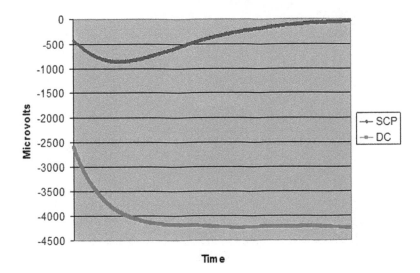

Plate 4 Comparison of SCP and DC signals for a 60-second epoch. The SCP signal (in blue) tends to stay near the baseline (zero value), while the DC signal stays at its full value, which exceeds −4,000 microvolts. The SCP signal reflects the negative deflection of the DC signal (in pink) and returns to baseline after the DC signal has stabilized.

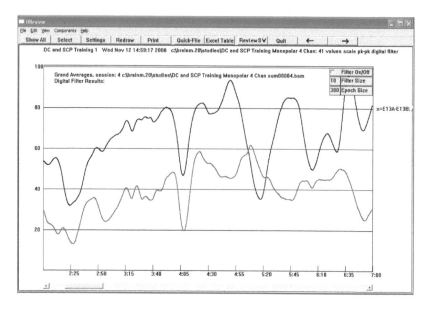

Plate 5 Comparison of F3 (black) and F4 (dark blue) SCP signals. The signals have periods of agreement, and also periods during which they are divergent and even out of phase.

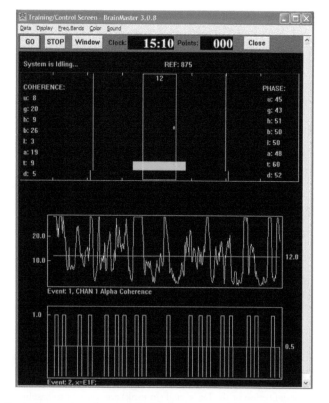

Plate 6 Typical operation of a neurofeedback system training coherence.

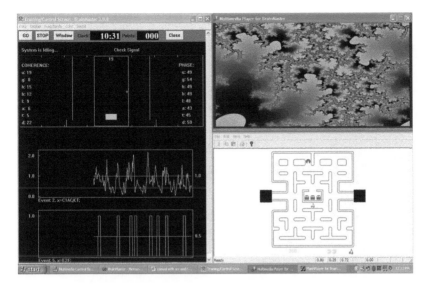

Plate 7 A set of neurofeedback screens. Control screen with graphic of metric (coherence), trend graph, and event markers indicating meeting of criterion (left). Animation of fractal display, and game screen showing rewards to trainee (right).

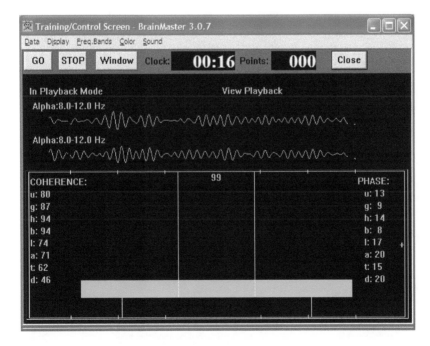

Plate 8 A control screen showing two filtered waveforms in the alpha band and their simultaneous coherence estimate.

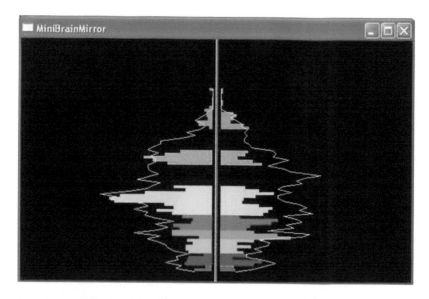

Plate 9 An EEG spectral display of two channels, showing the features relevant to the concurrent estimate of spectral correlation coefficient (SCC). The measurement answers the question "How similar (symmetrical) is the shape of the spectral amplitude of the two channels in a particular band?"

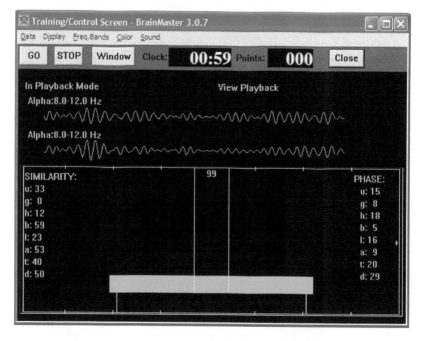

Plate 10 Control screen showing two signals, and their synchrony measure.

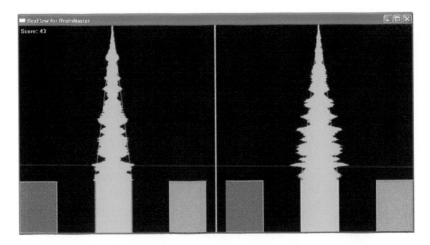

Plate 11 Control screen showing two amplitude envelopes, reflecting the information used to calculate comodulation.

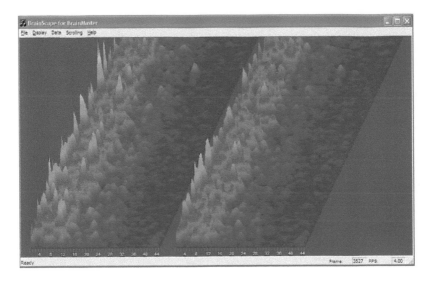

Plate 12 Fz and Cz in standard two-channel mode.

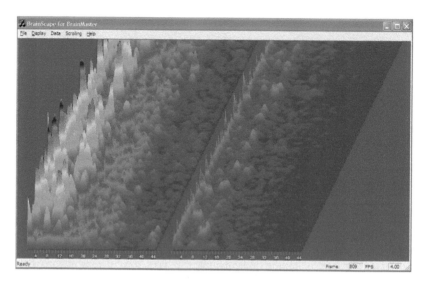

Plate 13 Fz and Cz in sum/difference channel mode.

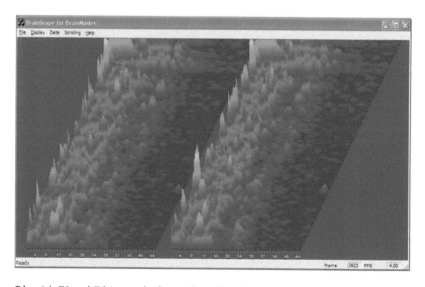

Plate 14 F3 and F4 in standard two-channel mode.

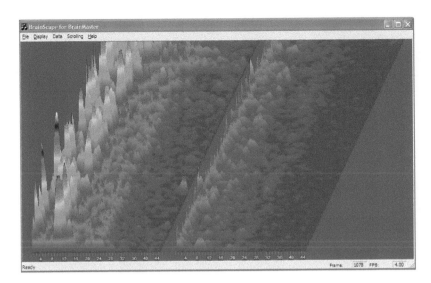

Plate 15 F3 and F4 in sum/difference channel mode.

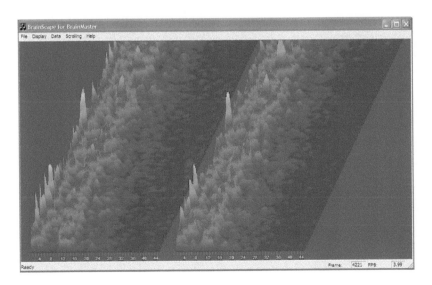

Plate 16 C3 and C4 in standard two-channel mode.

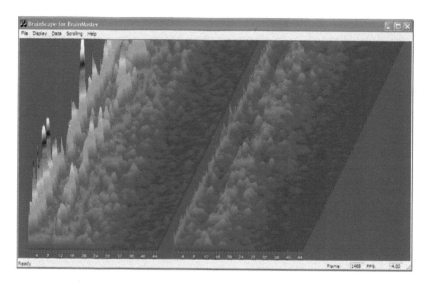

Plate 17 C3 and C4 in sum/difference channel mode.

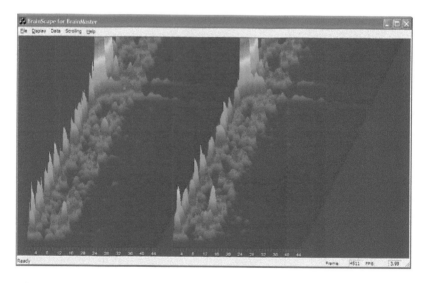

Plate 18 P3 and P4 in standard two-channel mode.

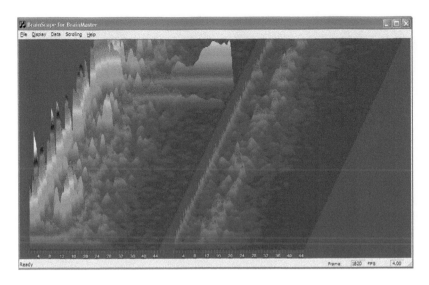

Plate 19 P3 and P4 in sum/difference channel mode.

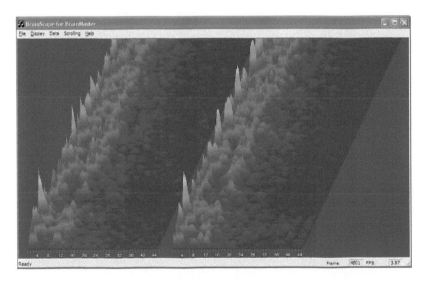

Plate 20 T3 and T4 in standard two-channel mode.

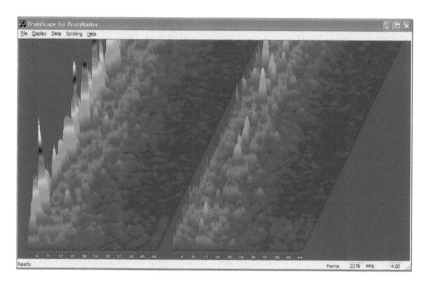

Plate 21 T3 and T4 in sum/difference channel mode.

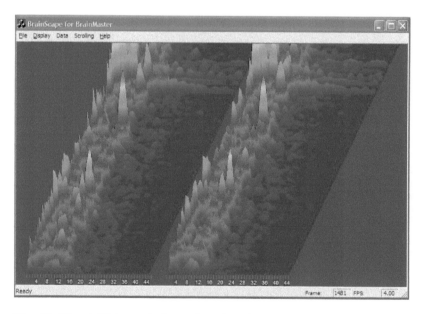

Plate 22 O1 and O2 in standard two-channel mode.

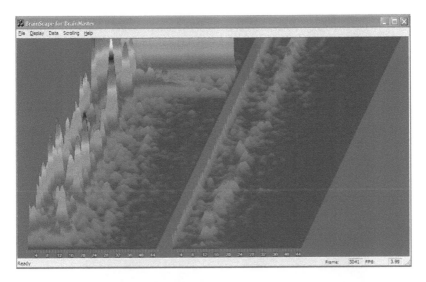

Plate 23 O1 and O2 in sum/difference channel mode.

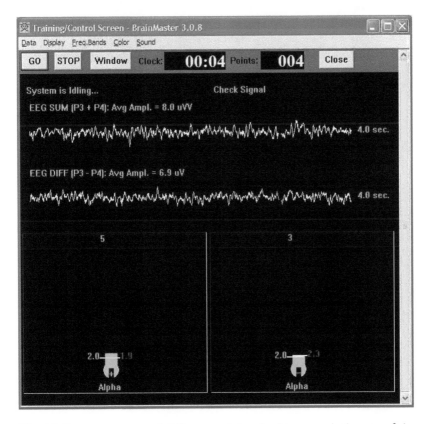

Plate 24 One-person sum and difference training. In this protocol, the sum of the channels is reinforced, while the difference is inhibited.

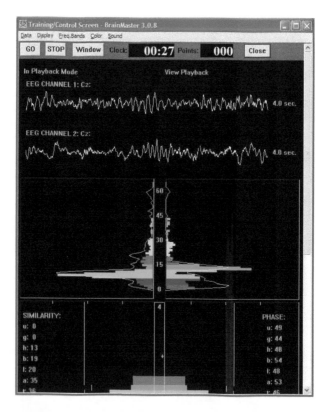

Plate 25 Training screen from two-person one-channel training, showing two individual EEGs being displayed and trained simultaneously. One person is using channel 1 and the other person is using channel 2. This trains them to synchronize their EEG waves to each other.

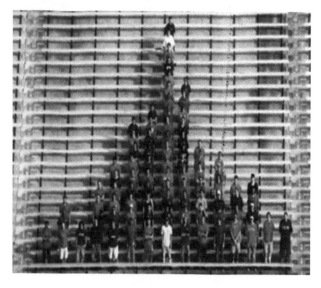

Plate 26 A population distribution of height among male athletes.

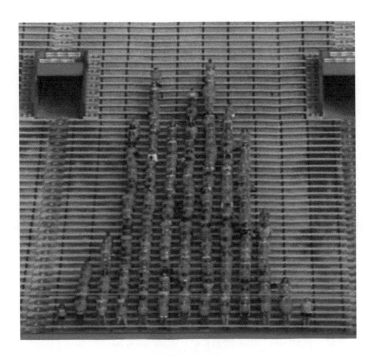

Plate 27 A population distribution of height among female athletes.

Training/Control Screen - BrainMaster 3.0.3

Data Display Freq.Bands Color Sound

| GO | STOP | Window | Clock: 19:26 | Points: 000 | Close |

System is Idling...   Check Signal

SITES: F3 F4 (EO)	Abs	Rel	Rat/T	Rat/A	Rat/B	Rat/G
Delta (1.0-4.0)	-0.5	-0.7	-0.4	-0.4	-0.4	-0.4
Theta (4.0-8.0)	-0.0	-0.1		-0.3	-0.3	-0.3
Alpha (8.0-12.5)	-0.0	-0.1			-0.9	-0.9
Beta (12.5-25.5)	0.7	0.7				-1.0
Beta 1 (12.0-15.5)	0.8	0.8				
Beta 2 (15.0-18.0)	0.8	0.8				
Beta 3 (18.0-25.5)	0.6	0.6				
Gamma (25.5-30.5)	0.6	0.7				
Delta (1.0-4.0)	-0.7	-0.9	-0.5	-0.5	-0.5	-0.5
Theta (4.0-8.0)	0.0	-0.0		-0.4	-0.4	-0.4
Alpha (8.0-12.5)	-0.1	-0.2			-1.0	-1.0
Beta (12.5-25.5)	0.6	0.7				-1.1
Beta 1 (12.0-15.5)	0.9	0.9				
Beta 2 (15.0-18.0)	0.6	0.7				
Beta 3 (18.0-25.5)	0.6	0.6				
Gamma (25.5-30.5)	0.7	0.7				

	Asymmetry	Coherence	Phase Difference
Delta (1.0-4.0)	0.2	-1.3	1.5
Theta (4.0-8.0)	-0.0	-1.7	1.3
Alpha (8.0-12.5)	0.1	-1.6	1.4
Beta (12.5-25.5)	0.0	-1.6	0.8
Beta 1 (12.0-15.5)	-0.0	-0.9	0.7
Beta 2 (15.0-18.0)	0.1	-1.0	1.0
Beta 3 (18.0-25.5)	0.0	-1.0	0.9
Gamma (25.5-30.5)	-0.0	-1.0	0.7

Plate 28 Live z-scores, two channels (76 targets): 26 × 2 + 24 = 76 (52 power, 24 connectivity).

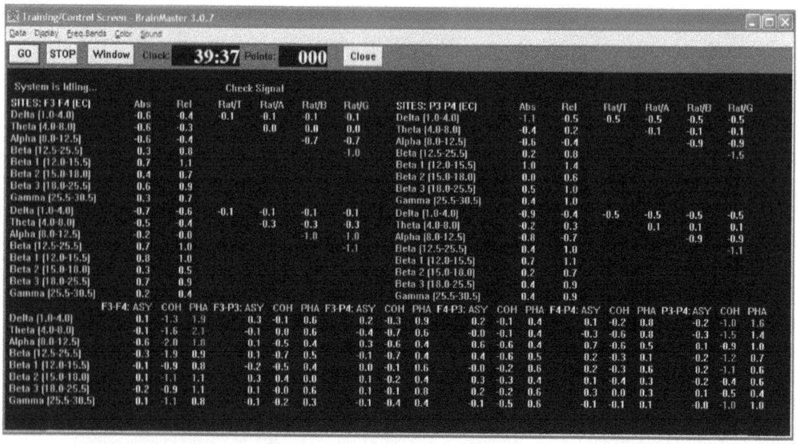

Plate 29 Live z-scores, four channels: $26 \times 4 + 24 \times 6 = 248$ (104 power, 144 connectivity).

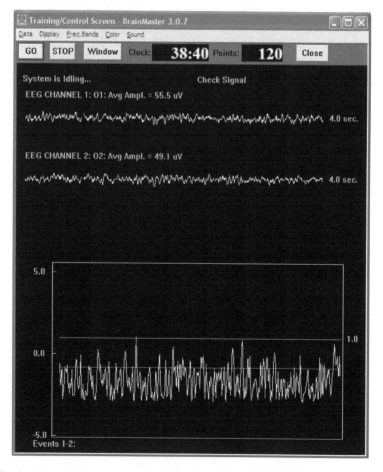

Plate 30 Z-score coherence range training.

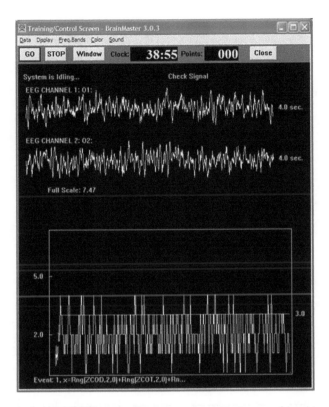

Plate 31 Live z-score training using four targets, in which the reward is achieved when all four variables are within their target range.

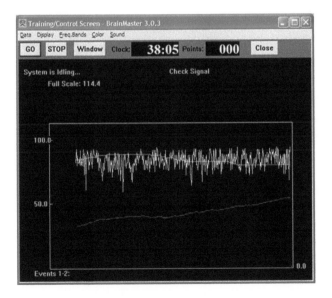

Plate 32 Multivariate proportional z-score feedback, showing the effect of varying the reward criterion. As the condition is relaxed so that a smaller percentage of z-scores can earn a reward, the reward rate increases.

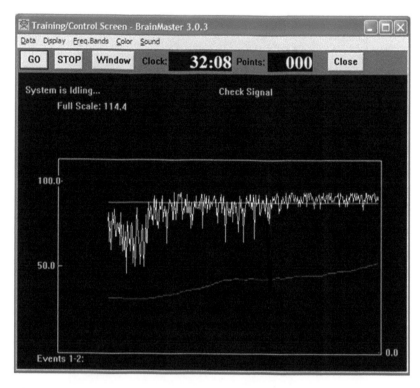

Plate 33 Multivariate proportional z-score feedback, showing the effect of varying the target size. As the target size is widened so that a larger percentage of z-scores can fit within the targets, the reward rate increases.

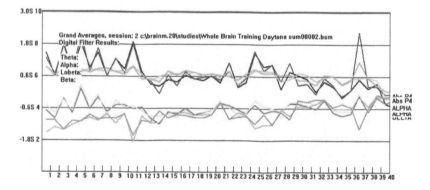

Plate 34 Individual z-score changes from a single 40-minute session.

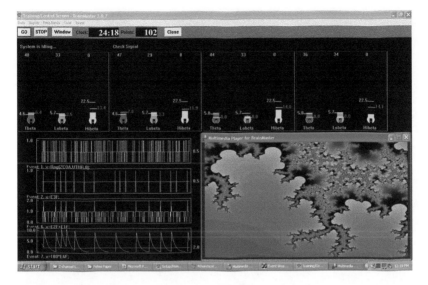

Plate 35 Combined z-score and traditional training.

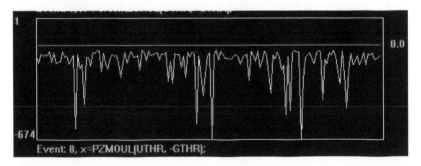

Plate 36 PZMO—"PZ Motive"—"percentage of z-score movement."

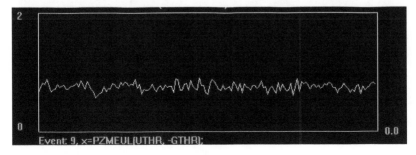

Plate 37 PZME—"PZ Mean" or "PZ Measure."

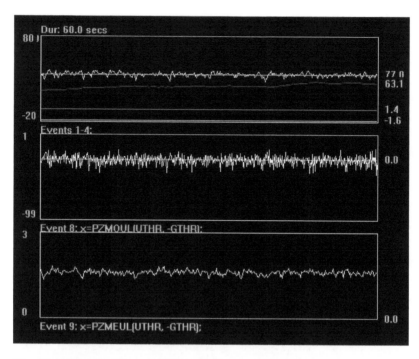

Plate 38 PZOK, PZMO, and PZME during a training session.

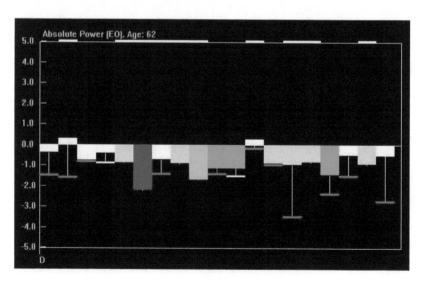

Plate 39 Z-Bars for absolute power during a training session.

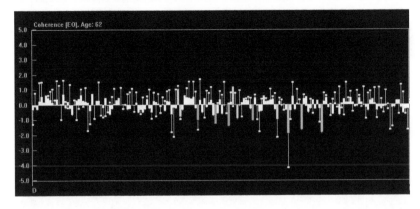

Plate 40 192 coherence z-scores shown from 19 channels.

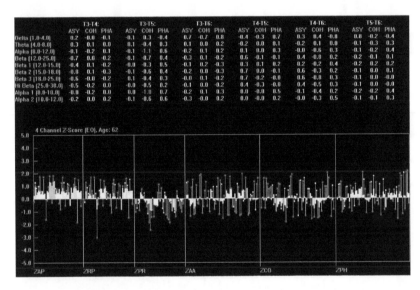

Plate 41 Simultaneous live z-score text and bars display, showing deviations in coherence between two particular sites.

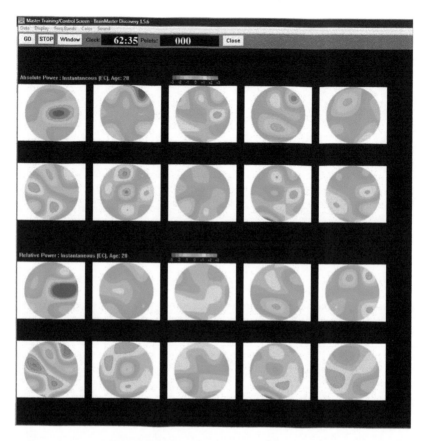

Plate 42 Live maps of z-scores for assessment and training.

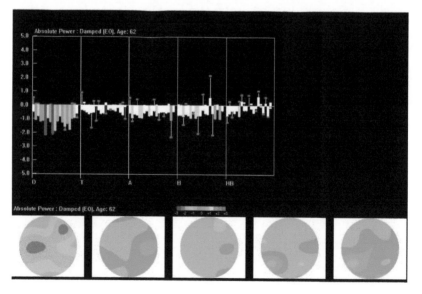

Plate 43 Simultaneous Z-Bars and Z-Maps during a live training session.

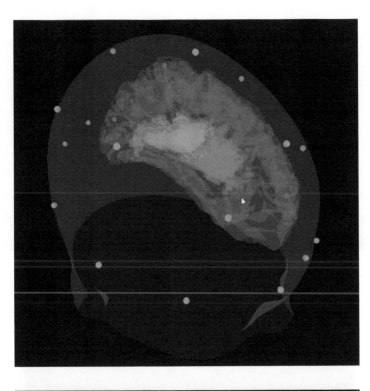

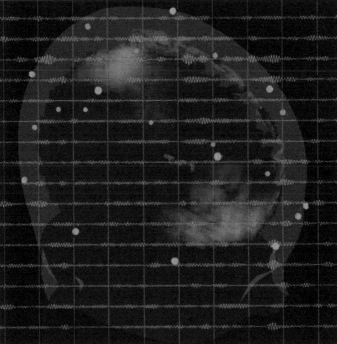

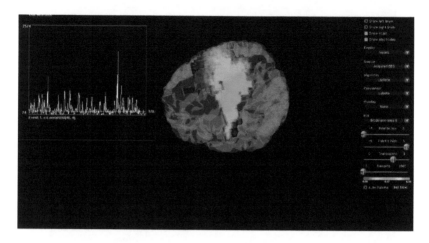

Plate 46 Illustration of live sLORETA power training, of Brodmann Area 4. The graph shows the total power in this band, in the component band being trained (12–20 Hz). Courtesy of Dr. N. Schnepel.

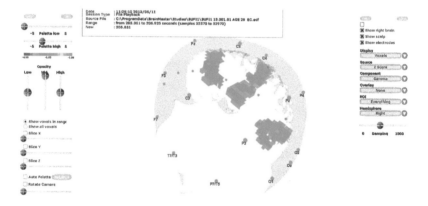

Plate 47 Illustration of a functional hub imaged using sLORETA z-scores. The regions which show high levels of gamma (35–50 Hz) include the occipital cortex, the sensory strip, and the ventromedial frontal cortex.

Plate 44 *(facing page, top)* sLORETA (Standardized Low-Resolution Electromagnetic Tomography) image of the beta activity in the cingulate gyrus, imaged in the form of current-source density (CSD). The gradient of activity from anterior to posterior is evident, showing that the anterior and posterior regions are more active than the central region.

Plate 45 *(facing page, bottom)* sLORETA image of the beta activity in the cortex of a client with anxiety and depression. The excess activity in the right dorsolateral frontal lobe is reflective of a negative mood, while the excess activity in the left parietal area likely reflects ruminating thoughts, possibly related to the client's self-image.

8

USE OF LIVE Z-SCORES

The use of live z-scores is a relatively recent development in EEG biofeedback. It takes advantage of the statistical concept of a normal distribution to convert any measurement into a z-score, which is a measure of distance from a target value. This value is generally a mean taken from a population, thus representing a target that is "normal." However, this is not a necessary condition, and it is possible to do live z-score training with various targets, besides those that represent the center of a population distribution.

The technical underpinnings of live z-score training were described by Thatcher (2008), who described how an EEG database can be used to derive target values and produce useful scores in real time. This technique takes advantage of joint time-frequency analysis (JTFA) as the means to extract short-term variations in target values, and convert them to useful means and standard deviations. Implementation of live z-score training had to wait until computers with sufficient capability, and software with sufficient flexibility, could be introduced.

Practical training using live z-scores was first reported by Collura et al. (2008), and has become an important element in modern neurofeedback. Before live z-scores, practitioners had to know the specific target values of each complement, and program this into the system. With the introduction of live z-scores, however, any EEG metric could be reduced to a z-score and trained in a desired direction.

Initial reports of clinical results with live z-scores have used a normative database based on a population of normal individuals. The advantage of this approach is that the targets are of a documented and well-defined nature, and reliably reflect the normal range of functioning of the human brain. While this has provided a strong foundation and significant clinical results, emerging methods are using alternative references to provide greater possibilities for individualized training, as well as for specific purposes.

When used in the context of normative training, z-scores provide a means to understand and employ population information and use it for individual assessment and training. However, although live z-score training originated using population statistics, we shall see that its application value does not depend on specifically using population data. Live z-score training is a structured method that can be applied to any measurement, and that can use targets derived from virtually any metric.

While live z-score training is a general approach, there are differences with regard to how variables are used, how feedback is presented, and the likely clinical outcome. In its simplest form, a single z-score can be used to define a target or target range. If it is used to train alpha, for example, it amounts to no more than a pair of thresholds whose values are looked up in a table based upon age, site, and eyes condition. This is of particular benefit when doing connectivity training, for which the use of a range is very important. However, it does not provide any form of systems training that cannot be achieved with conventional methods, albeit with somewhat less work. In order to fully exploit the potential of live z-score training, it is important to train multiple z-scores, and to develop the protocol approach in an intuitive and evidence-based manner.

In our work, we quickly moved into a more complex, yet intuitively simple, way of using multiple (hundreds of) z-scores in the training (Collura and Mrklas, 2008). One of our unique developments was the provision of "proportional" feedback reflecting "how well" the training was doing, rather than a simple on/off feedback signal. It was found that using this more complex information, as well as generalizing it to four channels, provided a key level of functionality that met with broad clinical acceptance. The first major deviation from simple z-score training that will be described is the use of various "multivariate proportional" feedback mechanisms that provide the trainee with particularly rich information. The second deviation that will be described is the move away from statistically based population norms and toward individualized training "templates" that represent real or hypothetic individual EEG profiles. The addition of template-based training targets to multivariate live z-score training provides a uniquely powerful and flexible platform for QEEG-based brainwave "shaping," not just normalization.

Historically, the references for live z-score training have been population statistics intended to reflect normal brain function. Statistical sampling and normalization techniques have been used to ensure that the resulting scores reflected normal ranges. When used for neurofeedback, these normative targets provide reinforcement when appropriate combinations of z-scores fall within predefined ranges of normal. This approach has demonstrated validity and clinical value as a basis for clinical neurofeedback. Positive results have been reported in single subject case reports (Collura et al., 2010) and in at least one controlled study (Festa et al., 2009). The general observation is that when clinical cases show EEG abnormalities, live z-score training can effectively lead toward normalization of the QEEG, along with symptomatic improvement.

Several issues arise with the use of a normative standard. The first is "Why should everyone of a given age have the same optimal EEG?"

Individual differences can be profound and should surely play a part in the neurofeedback protocol design. Second, there is the potential for reinforcing changes in EEG parameters that are not in the "normal" range, but are there for a reason. These will include two main categories: (1) peak performance or optimal functioning characteristic; and (2) coping and compensating mechanisms. These will be described in greater detail once we have covered the basic concepts of live z-score training.

Our approach to addressing the issues of individual signatures, peak performance characteristics, and coping mechanisms is to use a particular method that allows a certain percentage of "outliers" to remain outside the training range, even while the trainee receives reinforcement. Thus, it is possible to retain deviant z-scores in the EEG while still undergoing operant training and learning to shape the EEG towards normal values.

However, the fact remains that no individual, in fact, has all entirely zero z-scores. Rather, this reference reflects a fictitious individual. One of the limitations of using standardized normal z-score targets is that the individuals who belong, say, at 1 or 1.2 standard deviations as part of their individual profile will nonetheless be trained toward a target that, for them, is a deviation from their "normal." Indeed, any individual from the original sample, even if trained using the very database to which they contributed EEG, would be trained away from their normal state toward the population mean.

The basic idea behind z-score training is rather simple. For any EEG component, a target consists of a target value and a standard deviation. The target value and deviation can be different for each complement, and can depend on factors such as age, site location, and eyes condition or task condition. All that is really needed for z-score training is a target and a range to compare with the current measurement. For historical reasons, there is a tendency to think of the targets as coming from a database, particularly a database of normals. However, there is no reason that the targets must be from such a source, and any target value and range can be used to convert a measurement into a z-score.

Whatever the source of the z-score target, it ultimately consists of simply a mean and a standard deviation for any derived value. Given these two values, it is possible to convert any measurement into a z-score simply by applying the familiar formula:

$$z = \frac{x - \mu}{\sigma}$$

Or, in more familiar terms:

$$z\text{-score} = \frac{\text{measurement} - \text{mean}}{\text{stdev}}$$

The conceptual interpretation of a z-score is straightforward. Regardless of the origin of the mean and standard deviation used, the z-score is simply a measure of how many standard deviations the measurement is from the mean. A positive z-score indicates that the value is higher than the mean, and a negative z-score indicates that the value is lower. Z-scores can be computed for virtually any relevant variables. In neural feedback, the most common values are magnitude, referred to as power, relative power, power or magnitude ratios, and connectivity metrics such as coherence or phase. Asymmetry can also be used as an indicator of relative activation.

The values used in live z-score training are of necessity the same or similar two metrics that are familiar in quantitative EEG work. This is one of the reasons that targets have historically been based upon normative data. It is useful to look at an easily understood variable to illustrate z-scores and their use in assessment and training. The following example uses height as a relevant variable and demonstrates the population distribution of this measurement.

Color Plate 26 illustrates a population distribution of a basic parameter, that of height (Starr and Taggart, 2003, p. 89). All individuals of equal height (within 1 inch) are standing in the same column, with the shortest on the left and the tallest on the right. The mean height is clearly evident as the column in the middle of this symmetric bell curve. The standard deviation, of approximately 3 inches, is evident in the spread of this curve.

Color Plate 27 represents the same data for female athletes instead of males. In this case, the mean is different, and the standard deviation is also visibly different. There is clearly a tendency for the female heights to be more broadly distributed, with less of a pronounced peak in the middle. This will be reflected in a different standard deviation. In this example, gender is an important factor in establishing norms for height. Which factors are important for EEG is a different matter. Generally, age is considered, as is the condition of eyes open or eyes closed. Some EEG databases also include one or more task conditions.

Aside from the conditions and grouping factors, the EEG variables that are to be evaluated must also be chosen. The most common values are absolute power and relative power, with other derivative measures, such as power ratios and asymmetry, as well as connectivity-based measures.

While this example provides a clear picture of population z-scores, it does not lead directly to the conclusion that these scores are useful for operant training. Height, for example, is not a variable that is particularly amenable to operant training, so the logic extending population data to feedback training must be made on grounds that appeal to functioning and self-regulation.

Neurofeedback in general, and live z-score training in particular, appeal to the notion of neuroplasticity, and the fact that the brain is a dynamically organized and reconfigurable system. Learning is a key element of this strategy, and it should be demonstrable that learning can occur, and that it is clinically relevant. It further needs to be clear that the use of a normative or any other reference is reasonable for the clinical application.

Some Important Conceptual Points Related to Z-Scores and Population Statistics

While a significant deviation from the norm is to be noted, and if it is correlated with a clinical "complaint" it should be addressed, it is by no means clear that the ideal value is "zero" for everyone. Indeed, the reason the bell curve exists is that there are individuals who "belong" at each and every value along the curve. In fact, it is possible that an individual may be at −0.7, for example, and they "should" be at +0.5, not 0.0. Or, it is possible that a client who is at 0.3 might actually need to be at 0.9, so that his or her preferred direction is away, not toward, the mean.

It is one thing to define a z-score and to compute it in real time, but it is another matter entirely to use it in practical neurofeedback. An initial observation is that a single z-score used as a target is simply the same target redefined. With the exception of the fact that the z-score is conveniently trained within a range, there is no difference in the feedback that the brain sees, whether the feedback is based upon a z-score or a raw score. The real strength of live z-score training arises when multiple z-scores are used. In this context, the brain is being provided with information about global

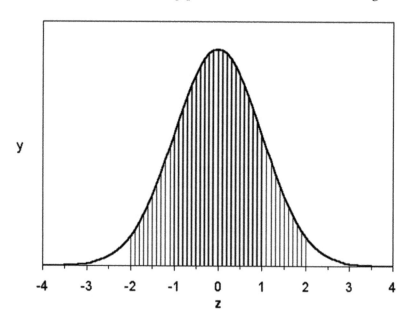

Figure 8.1 A typical normal "bell curve" with deviations expressed in z-scores.

Z-Score Ranges

- +/– 1 sigma:
  - Includes middle 68 percent of population.
  - From 16 percent to 84 percent points.
- +/– 2 sigma:
  - Includes middle 95 percent of population.
  - From 2 percent to 98 percent points.
- +/– 3 sigma:
  - Includes middles 99.8 percent of population.
  - From 0.1 percent to 99.99 percent points.
- +/– 4 sigma:
  - More likely from a different population (distribution).

function and normalization, and can be given more complex tasks to do. Using the metaphor of riding a bicycle, conventional neurofeedback with one, two, or three targets is a much simpler task, addressing some aspect of activation or relaxation. But when multiple z-scores are incorporated into the feedback, the brain is being provided with more information, including mutual activation, communication, and other global brain processes.

Instantaneous versus Static Z-Scores

When live z-scores are compared with the z-scores obtained from assessment summary data, there is a difference in the observed values. Generally, instantaneous z-scores will report smaller values, corresponding to a larger expected range (standard deviation). Thus, a client whose beta is 3 standard deviations large according to the summary report will typically show live z-scores in the range of 1.5 to 2.0 standard deviations.

Basically, it is very difficult for something to happen in the short term that is that unusual. However, when unusual behavior persists over longer periods of time, it becomes more unusual. A single "par" hole is not that unusual in golf, but a consistent string of them is what separates a mere pro from a champion golfer. Using this analogy, a live z-score is like the score on a single hole. If we consider a birdie to be +1, par to be zero, and a bogey to be –1, then these are the values possible on a single hole. Therefore, it is not possible generally to get a highly unusual score on a single hole. However, based upon 18 holes of performance, if a player manages to achieve 18 birdies, then his or her total score will be 18 points lower than par. This would be a very unlikely event. Therefore, an unusual result can be obtained by consistent achievement of less extreme results.

Typical Z-Scores Used in Neurofeedback

- Absolute power (10 bands per channel).
- Relative power (10 bands per channel).
- Power ratios (10 ratios per channel).
- Asymmetry (10 bands per path).
- Coherence (10 bands per path).
- Phase (10 bands per path).
- Based on age, eyes open/closed.

The common metrics used with live z-score training are summarized as follows. Absolute power is a measure of the size of each component, generally expressed in microvolts or microvolts squared. It reflects how much of the component is present. Relative power is the size of a component divided by the total power in the EEG. It reflects how much of the component is present, compared to all others. Power ratio is the size of a component divided by the size of another component. The most commonly used power ratio is the beta/theta ratio. Asymmetry is the size of a component at one location divided by the size at another location. It reflects the differential activation of different parts of the brain. An important example is the frontal left/right alpha asymmetry. Coherence is a measure of the amount of information shared between two sites, such as the alpha coherence that generally reflects the degree of uniform thalamo-cortical reverberation. Phase is a measure of the speed of information sharing between two sites, and is important to the assessment of information processing. See Color Plates 28 and 29.

Z-Score Targeting Strategies

- Train z-score(s) up or down:
  - Simple directional training.
- Train z-score(s) using Rng():
  - Set size and location of target(s).
- Train z-score(s) using percentZOK():
  - Set width of z-window via percentZOK (range).
  - Set percent floor as a threshold.
- Combine the above with other training (e.g. power training).

See Color Plate 30.

Use of "Range" Function

- Rng(VAR, RANGE, CENTER)
- = 1 if VAR is within RANGE of CENTER
- = 0 else
- Rng(BCOH, 10, 30)
  - 1 if beta coherence is within +/–10 of 30
- Rng(ZCOB, 2, 0)
  - 1 if beta coherence z score is within +/–2 of 0

See Color Plate 31.

Training with Multiple Ranges

- X = Rng(ZCOD, 2,0) + Rng(ZCOT, 2, 0), + Rng(ZCOA, 2, 0) + Rng(ZCOB, 2, 0)
- = 0 if no coherences are in range
- = 1 if 1 coherence is in range
- = 2 if 2 coherences are in range
- = 3 if 3 coherences are in range
- = 4 if all 4 coherences are in range
- Creates new training variable, target = 4

Multivariate Training—Percent ZOK

Operant conditioning using multiple z-scores employs certain specific mechanisms that underlie its efficacy and flexibility (Collura and Mrklas, 2008). The approach described here produces a feedback variable that is not simply an on/off response, but contains quantitative information regarding the state of the z-scores. John (2001) describes the set of z-scores as a multivariate space whose complex dimensions encode key brain functional parameters. By feeding back specific variables related to the distribution of z-scores, the trainee is provided with information that can be used in a complex guidance manner. Our motivation for training multivariate z-score parameters is based partly on this point of view. We envision the live z-scores as being essential indicators of brain dynamics, beyond their simple ability to indicate whether a value is within a certain statistical range. What is more important is the ability to feed back a complex and informative feedback that allows the brain to explore its internal state by making dynamic changes and experiencing the consequences.

The percentage of z-scores that fit within a predefined range is a metric that allows the trainee to grasp how similar his or her EEG is to a reference EEG. The specific z-scores that are included in the target range are not specified beforehand, only the percentage of scores that must fit. This provides an opportunity for learning that is relevant to the self-regulation of complex brain dynamics.

In using this multivariate approach, clinicians are faced with operational decisions, such as the size of the target range and the percentage of z-scores that must fall within the training targets in order to receive a reward. There are specific advantages and disadvantages to using relatively small or relatively large targets. When wide target ranges are used, and it is possible to fit most or all of the z-scores into the target range, then those scores that are differentially trained are, by definition, the most deviant. While this may seem reasonable, particularly when the deviant scores are contributing to the clinical issue, it raises an important question. It cannot be ensured that these most deviant scores are, in fact, the most relevant to normal brain processing. Indeed, these scores may and will likely include deviations due to artifact or related transient phenomena. If this is the case, then training the most deviant z-scores may amount to little more than suppressing artifact.

A typical simplistic live z-score protocol might include one or more z-scores and require all of them to fit within the target range. This is reasonable when a small number of highly relevant z-scores can be identified along with an appropriate range. One drawback of this approach is that z-scores that are not being monitored remain free to change during the training. Therefore, it is reasonable to look for a strategy that looks broadly at the z-scores and keeps them in check. A second drawback to using wide targets is that the z-scores that live well within this wide boundary are still free to vary. This variation has the disadvantage of possibly allowing z-scores that had been close to normal to deviate away from the normal range. Because the target area is relatively large, such deviations would not be detected unless the z-scores leave the target range.

In our multivariate work, we quickly moved to a scheme in which only a proportion of the z-scores needed to fall with in a target range. This allowed the ability to avoid simply training outliers, and was found to provide valuable feedback for clinical training.

The choice of target sizes represents two polar extremes when very narrow or very wide targets are considered. The value of each in learning can be understood by analogy to tests used in education. In early years, it can be common to give vocabulary spelling words to a child and expect essentially all of them to be done correctly. In this case, the task consists of relatively easy elements, all of which are expected to be correct. This situation is analogous to a very wide target, and the requirement that all z-scores conform. As one encounters high school level math, it may occur that the teacher will say "I will not deduct points for arithmetic mistakes." That is to say, the complex concepts are emphasized, while minor errors are neglected. This is similar to reducing the target size somewhat and allowing a certain set of outliers to be ignored. In more advanced education, one might encounter a very difficult technical subject in which the instructor is willing to pass any student who achieves 50 or 60 percent or more. I personally have been in physics courses where the professor actually said he would not deduct for simple algebra or even calculus mistakes. The point to be made here is that it is possible to achieve learning by looking critically at a subset of the performance, and allowing certain aspects of the performance to be ignored. In multivariate live z-score training, the client's brain is able to determine which variables remain outside the targets as a personal strategy.

One of the disadvantages of using a narrow target range and a percentage of z-scores is that now the outliers themselves become disregarded in the training. That is, if a variable remains outside the training range more or less continually, then its behavior has no effect on feedback. This consideration is one of the motivations for the derivative variables that will be described below.

- PercentZOK(RANGE)
  - Gives percent of z-scores within RANGE of 0
  - One channel: 26 z-scores total
  - Two channels: 76 z-scores total
  - Four channels: 248 z-scores total
- Value = 0 to 100
- Measure of "How Normal?"

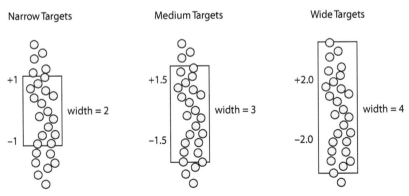

Figure 8.2 Live z-score multivariate proportional (MVP) feedback showing the effect of varying the target size for a population of z-scores.

Color Plate 32 shows the changes in the PZOK output as the percentage threshold is changed. When the percentage of z-scores required is reduced, then the percentage of time meeting criteria is seen to increase.

Color Plate 33 shows the changes in the PZOK output as the target size is changed. When the targets are widened, then the percentage of time meeting criteria is seen to increase. As this happens, the more deviant z-scores (outliers) are emphasized.

Results of Multivariate Live Z-Score Training

Figure 8.3 shows the difference between the variable distributions that are obtained by analyzing a single individual, as well as multiple individuals. When z-scores are computed from a sample value, they are based upon a distribution of this type.

What is the underlying mechanism that governs multivariate live z-score training? It is clear that this is an operant learning paradigm, but the question remains as to how the brain is dealing with the information provided. When beginning this work, there was concern that the brain might not be able to unravel the complex information being considered. It was likened to combing a tangle that offered no starting point.

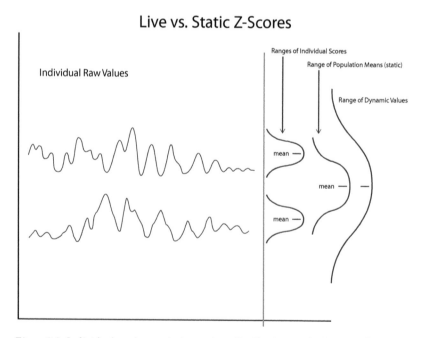

Figure 8.3 Individual and population value distributions, which are reflected in z-scores.

What has become evident through inspection of live training results and summary data is that the brain effectively undergoes a search strategy that can be described as a single-person gain. Nash (1950) described some important aspects of these gains and described the situation in which a player is able to manipulate one or more variables, and experience a result (Sethi, 2007). A Nash game proceeds when one or more players begin to manipulate variables and receive the payoff functions. In our example, the brain is the player and the brain function can be manipulated so as to produce differing z-scores.

A Nash equilibrium is said to occur when any change in any player variable results in a lower score. Therefore, if an individual's z-scores were all at their closest levels to the mean, then any alteration would lower their multivariate score. There is a tacit sense that in live z-score training, the goal is for the client to achieve something like this equilibrium. I do not entirely subscribe to this view, which is another motivation for the multivariate strategy described here. It is sufficient for the brain to implement a strategy that consistently produces high scores, consistent with the level of comfort and other criteria the brain is using to judge its performance.

An important aspect of Nash equilibria is the fact that many systems will have multiple stable equilibria. A local equilibrium point may exist into which the organism is essentially stock, but that does not reflect global optimization. The possibility of multiple Nash equilibria is a critical point in this context. It provides a model for understanding disk-regulated brain dynamics, in terms of being a suboptimal but local equilibrium point.

By introducing additional criteria for the brain to self-regulate, live z-score training presents the opportunity to escape local equilibria and to move toward more globally optimal states. This strategy is also evident in the game MindMaster, as illustrated in Figure 8.4. In this game, a player makes successive gases using colored pegs and is provided with feedback showing the success of each trial. By making successive changes and seeing the results, a player can ascertain the target configuration of colors and thus discover the solution. The analogy between this game and live z-score training was suggested by Rutter (2011) and described in more detail by Stoller (2011).

Color Plate 34 illustrates results from a single subject session of 40 minutes, during which this type of search and optimization strategy is evident.

Figure 8.5 shows the percentage of z-scores within the target range as a function of time over the same 40-minute session. The initial "hunting" behavior is evident during the first 10 minutes, after which the trainee reported that he was "getting it."

Based upon this understanding of brain operant training and a knowledge of specific human brain dynamics and parameters, it is possible to apply live z-score training to a variety of clinical situations. However, it should

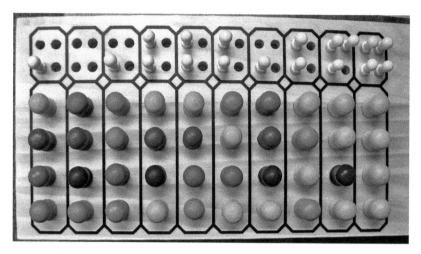

Figure 8.4 MindMaster.

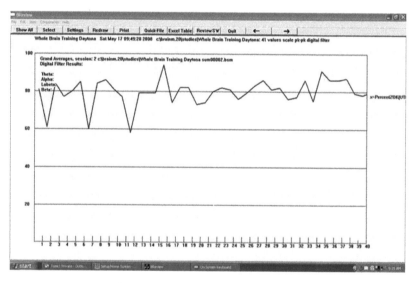

Figure 8.5 Perentage of z-scores within the target range over a 40-minute session.

be emphasized that live z-score training is not a panacea, and it is certainly not the case that one can apply censors indiscriminately and train everyone to the same targets.

There are various specific clinical situations in which multivariate live z-score training makes particular sense and has been found to be effective.

166

Normalize Using Z-Scores

- Excessive frontal slowing.
- Excessive beta or high beta.
- Hyper-coherence, not left hemisphere (F3-P3).
- Hypo-coherence, not central (C3-C4).
- Localized (focal) excess or deficit.

Coping/Compensating Z-Scores

- Diffuse low alpha:
  - chronic pain (barrier).
- Diffuse high alpha:
  - chronic anxiety coping mechanism.
- Posterior asymmetries:
  - PTSD, stress coping, cognitive dissonance.

Peak Performance Z-Scores

- Left hemispheric hyper-coherence (F3-P3).
- Central intra-hemispheric hypo-coherence (C3-C4).
- "Excess" SMR C4.
- "Excess" posterior alpha.
- "Fast" posterior alpha.
- Note: normalization can be avoided by keeping EEG sensors away from affected sites.

Summary: Live Z-Score Neurofeedback

- New method using normative data.
- Comprehensive whole-head approach.
- Normalizes both activation and connectivity.
- Multiple targeting and biasing capability.
- Consistent with QEEG and phenotype approaches.
- Provides brain with complex information.
- Simple training format.
- Effective for assessment and training.

Phenotypes and Z-Scores

- Many phenotypes "map" to live z-scores:
  - diffuse slow;
  - focal abnormalities, not epileptiform;
  - mixed fast and slow;
  - frontal lobe disturbances—excess slow;
  - frontal asymmetries;
  - excess temporal lobe alpha;
  - spindling excessive beta;
  - generally low magnitudes;
  - persistent alpha; and
  - diffuse alpha deficit.
  - Exceptions:
  - "epileptiform" (requires visual inspection of EEG wave-forms);
  - faster alpha variants, not low voltage (requires live z-score for peak frequency);
  - many phenotypes can be addressed via LZT training;
  - inhibits, rewards referenced to normal population or biased for enhance/inhibit;
  - phenotypes do not (currently) consider connectivity deviations;
  - hypo-coherent intra-hemispheric (L or R);
  - hyper-coherent inter-hemispheric (e.g. frontal); and
  - diffuse coherence/phase abnormalities.

Color Plate 35 shows a control screen using a combination of traditional and live z-Score training. In this approach, both amplitude-based criteria and z-score criteria are applied. The z-score criteria ensure that coherences are within a normal range for the involved sites. The amplitude criteria are set to enhance a midrange band (SMR) while inhibiting theta and high beta. The combination of criteria provides a brief reinforcement using the video, followed by a refractory period.

Another variation on this approach is the use of multiple thresholds with live z-scores. It is possible to set thresholds in terms of the percentage of z-scores meeting criteria, so that one sound is heard for 60 percent, another for 70 percent, another for 80 percent, and so on. As a result, the client receives a type of multilevel feedback in which the feedback variable is not the size of a value, but is the number of z-scores that meet the condition.

We have described LZT methods that provide multivariate proportional (MVP) variables for use in training. MVP variables are continuous, proportional values that are used in training in the same ways that conventional values, such as absolute power, relative power, or raw coherence values, have been used in the past. MVP variables can provide complex yet intuitively simple measurements and client results that are rapid, concise, and lasting. Other approaches to live z-score training produce an "on/off" response, depending on whether one or more z-scores are within a range. Thus, the brain is provided with information that tells it whether or not it meets a condition, but does not provide any proportional or "how much" information to the trainee. This may limit the brain's ability to learn and respond to salient EEG parameters. Also, such methods do not lend themselves to tuning the training beyond setting the target sizes. Multivariate methods produce quantitative variables that are not simply "yes/no," but provide real-time, proportional feedback that can be used for sounds, videos, games, or other feedback methods that respond to either "on/off," "how much," or a combination of such control variables.

Starting with the "PZOK" training method, it has been possible to develop a family of training variables that intuitively incorporate any or all of the z-scores and turn them into a single proportional variable (Collura and Mrklas, 2008). With these variables, any combination of channels, parameters (absolute power, relative power, power ratios, coherence, phase, asymmetry), or frequency components (e.g. delta, theta, etc.) can be trained. Regardless of the number of channels or parameters chosen, this variable always has the same meaning. It is the "percent of z-scores that are within the target limits." It has a maximum value of 100 (100 percent "normal") that continuously varies in time, and is useful both for training and for assessing the overall condition of the client. This method has been proven since 2005, and has been published in a variety of peer-reviewed journals, books, and industry publications (Collura et al. 2008; 2010).

This provides the ability to dynamically change the difficulty of the training on multiple levels in real time without interrupting training. This is analogous to being able to adjust the throttle, choke, etc. of a vehicle while it is in motion, which is an essential element of clinical application. With the PZOK method, clinicians commonly adjust the size of the training window, and also the percentage of z-scores that are required to be met in order to obtain a reward. This was a non-obvious yet critical step in the evolution of BrainMaster's exclusive LZT technology.

PZOK provides a uniquely flexible and powerful approach to adjusting training conditions, particularly in real time. By alternating changes in either the target sizes or the percentage of z-score required, the clinician can adjust the difficulty level of the training, as well the distribution of the z-scores that are being trained. For example, requiring a large percentage of the z-scores to fit within a wide range emphasizes the "outliers" while ignoring smaller z-scores. On the other hand, requiring a small percentage of the z-scores to fit within a narrow target can provide a "challenge" form of training that emphasizes mid-range values while ignoring outliers. This latter method can, for example, leave the brain free to exhibit abnormalities that are compensating or coping mechanisms that persist, and allow the brain to formulate its own self-regulation strategy. The ability to ignore outliers is, at times, an important benefit. At other times, it is desirable to focus on outliers. The new metrics in the "Z-Plus" package address the outliers in new ways that increase the power and flexibility of PZOK training.

PZOK has been shown to have significant clinical value, and it can also be combined with other methods. A number of our protocols combine LZT training with "biased" training, such as alpha up, theta down, or other types of protocols. The combined protocols provide the same simple feedback to the client, but also guide his or her brain in a particular direction desired by the clinician. All new "Z-Plus" based designs can also be combined with traditional training, as the clinical sees fit.

"Z-Plus" extensions are designed to extend and reinforce the PZOK approach. Rather than changing or replacing the PZOK methods, the new software and displays provide additional information, flexibility, and direction for LZT training.

We first review PZOK in detail, and then introduce the new metrics, PZMO and PZME.

PZOK means "percentage of all trained z-scores that fall within a given target range."

PZOK provides an overall assessment of "how normal" by counting how many of the z-scores fit within the desired target range. The exact position of the z-scores is not important, only whether or not they are within the target limits. PZOK is useful as a real-time training variable. The clinician sets the size of the targets, and also the percent of z-scores required to achieve reward, and the client learns when the PZOK value exceeds the percentage target. It was found important to allow the percentage target to go below 100 percent in order to avoid simply training on "outliers" all the time.

PZOK has the following behavior:

- Minimum value: 0 ("no z-scores are within range").
- Maximum value: 100 ("all z-scores are within range").
- Intermediate values: 0 to 100 ("what percentage of z-scores are within range").
- Limiting behavior:
  - PZOK with very small target limits: not useful—PZOK becomes very small, even zero (no z-scores within range).

170

- PZOK with very large target limits: not useful—PZOK will always be 100 with very wide limits (all z-scores within range).
- Strengths of PZOK:
  - With any percentage less than 100 percent, PZOK allows you to ignore outliers (allows for coping or compensating mechanisms).
  - Adjustable target sizes to set difficulty of targets.
  - Adjustable percent of targets setting sets total reward rate.
  - Alternates between "challenge" and "easy" conditions for dynamic control of feedback, training of flexibility.
- Weaknesses of PZOK:
  - When targets are small, outliers are ignored, might deviate further.
  - When targets are wide, inner values are ignored, even if they move toward abnormal.
  - Only counts whether values are in range, does not analyze their size.
  - Treats all z-scores the same, no weighting at this time.
  - Requires attention to target limits, which should generally be adjusted.

Z-Plus: A Next Generation of LZT Training Software

When introduced, PZOK was met with skepticism by some in the industry, while it was adopted and studied by others. Many of the initial objections were categorical (i.e. they addressed concepts or issues, not realities). Some objections reflected a lack of grasp, rather than a critical understanding of the methods. Five years of clinical application and publication have resolved the categorical objections, while showing that we do need to address issues such as how to treat outliers and how to give different types of z-scores different weights. Nonetheless, over time, it has become clear that PZOK is uniquely capable of delivering meaningful and useful feedback in a wide range of client situations. Most of the initial objections to PZOK have been found insignificant, as the refinement and use of the technique has evolved into a sound clinical approach. The existing PZOK technology is entirely consistent with principles of operant conditioning, learning, and physiological adaptation. All that is special is that the information fed back (the "operant") is a complex yet useful reflection of brain state. As the industry continues to look to BrainMaster for leadership, we introduce a new series of functions that extend the intuition and usefulness of PZOK into new dimensions, the dimensions of "Z-Plus."

Based on our experience and analysis, we introduced two new families of metrics, plus additional displays, combined into the "Z-Plus" software option. "Z-Plus" is entirely consistent with, and extends, the existing LZT software, designs, and methods that have been proven over the last five years. Like PZOK, the new functions are also accessible as "UL" versions that use different upper and lower limits. The new functions are incorporated using the Event Wizard, and no new control panels or settings are required. This provides complete flexibility in how they are used, and does not require the clinician to stop using PZOK or to choose between methods. All metrics are always available, and protocols can be designed as desired, combining old with new as desired.

As will be seen below, one interesting aspect of the new metrics is that while they are useful with various target sizes, they are particularly useful with very small, even zero, target sizes. When target size is zero, the new metrics incorporate all z-scores into the calculation, providing true indicators of total system state and state change, and no z-scores will be ignored. This provides the ability to account for both outliers and intermediate z-scores without ignoring any z-scores.

PZMO (Color Plate 36) provides an overall assessment of the instantaneous movement (change) of all z-scores that are outside the specified range. Z-scores that are within the target range are ignored. PZMO uses concepts from physics to introduce the idea of "momentum" of the z-scores, which reflects their " velocity," direction," and also a weighting factor suggesting their "mass." It is not necessary to weigh all z-scores the same. With PZMO, it is possible to weigh different z-scores differently, providing an additional dimension of flexibility and control. PZMO is a z-score "motivator" and reflects the net z-score motion. PZMO takes into account not just the direction (towards or away from normal), but also the amount of movement (a little or a lot), and the weight of each z-score ("lightweight" versus "heavy"). PZMO can be positive or negative, and reflects the total change in "momentum" of all z-scores. When it is positive, then the net movement of all z-scores outside the target range is inward, toward normal. When it is negative, then the net movement of the outlying z-scores is outward, away from normal. Thus, PZMO provides an instantaneous indicator of the *change* in the z-scores, indicating the brain's immediate tendency toward normalization, or toward disregulation. Technically, PZMO is the instantaneous change in the total "momentum" of the system, as defined in physics.

PZMO is intended to be used in addition to PZOK. Existing protocols do not have to be changed, only extended (with a single Event Wizard event) to incorporate the PZMO data. Typically, when PZMO is above some positive threshold, the client will receive a bell, tone, or other reward. This provides an additional, highly dynamic reward (think of it as a "gold star") when the client moves in the right direction.

PZMO incorporates useful and intuitive concepts from astronomy, particularly celestial mechanics. The client is learning about his or her "gravitational potential," which is the tendency toward normalization. The training limit region is like a star and the outlying z-scores are like planets. Ideally, z-scores tend to move inward, to be captured by the sun. If all planets are in the sun, then all z-scores are within range, and the client's EEG is deemed normal. If a client can increase his or her "potential," then z-scores will normalize more directly and consistently. The training limits define a "capture area" similar to the event horizon of a black hole. Once z-scores go inside the boundaries, they disappear (are ignored). Only the z-scores moving outside the boundaries (the orbiting z-scores, if you will) are incorporated into PZMO. Thus, PZMO captures the tendency for z-scores ("planets") to move toward, not away from, their "sun." This puts the training into a highly visual and dynamic context. This informs the clinician, as well as the client, as to what is happening, and to what extent, in the complex dynamic "z-solar system" of the brain.

PZMO does not provide an overall assessment of "how normal" in the way that PZOK does. If all z-scores are within the target range and none are outside, then there is no net movement to reflect, and PZMO will be zero. At that point, PZOK would be 100. Thus, PZMO gives a rapid, intuitive indication of the direction of change and has higher resolution and responsiveness than PZOK. As an analogy, it is somewhat like adding a tachometer, or actually an accelerometer, to a car dashboard so that you can see how rapidly, and in what direction, your velocity is changing. It is also like a dieter monitoring the change in his or her weight every day as an indication of how the diet is working. PZMO introduces the idea that z-scores closer to normal have lower "potential energy," and that the client's brain has a natural tendency to normalize. The normal brain is a "rest state," toward which the brain should naturally move. Abnormalities require the brain to expend energy, and can be normalized as the brain relaxes and brain dynamics settle into an optimal state.

PZMO can be thought of as conveying "motion," "movement," "momentum," or related concepts to LZT training. It introduces concepts that derive from physics, including gravity, velocity, acceleration, and dynamic behavior. Using PZMO, the practitioner can begin to think of z-scores as objects that have mass, direction, even intention. The intuitive view of PZMO is that if it is 100, then that is the maximum inward movement, and thus all the outlying z-scores have just moved inside the target limits. If PZMO is 0, then there is no net movement (i.e. there is just as much inward movement as outward movement). If PZMO is negative, then the z-scores are in general moving outward. For example, if a client clenches his or her teeth, PZMO will immediately become a very large negative number. When he or she relaxes, it will become a very large positive number. In the long run, if there is net improvement, PZMO will be positive more often than it is negative. The client should get a reward when PZMO is sufficiently positive, for example above 10, which would mean that the net motion of the outliers is to move 10 percent of the distance toward normal. PZMO will not generally be positive all the time, as the z-scores in their typical patterns of movement simply cannot always be moving toward normal all the time.

PZMO emphasizes variability and dynamic change. It is analogous to a financial derivative that focuses on the change of a system, not simply its current state. As such, it has the potential to "leverage" LZT training by providing highly accurate information relating to dynamic change, and delivering it to the client. Again, PZMO is not intended to replace PZOK; it is intended to be used as a supplemental training or assessment variable. If the client receives an extra reward every time there is a significant inward movement, then he or she will learn that skill as well, and tend to reinforce the process of normalization, not just the state of being "more normal."

As an example of the use of PZMO, you might use the following event: If "x = PZMO(1);" IS GREATER THAN 10 THEN (play wav file).

This event would allow the user to hear a "beep" every time he or she achieved a 10 percent movement toward normal during the session. He or she would hear the reward whenever the z-scores had significant improvement, even if PZOK was not yet above the target percentage. This thus rewards improvement in the right direction, regardless of the current state. This motivating feedback is a significant addition to watching the PZOK variable rise and fall; it allows the client to know when he or she is moving in the right direction.

PZMO has the following behavior:

- Minimum value: negative value, unlimited ("z-scores are moving outward").
- Maximum value: 100 ("all z-scores have just moved within the target range").
- Intermediate values: typically −100 to +100: ("what is the overall motion toward or away from normal").
- Limiting behavior:
  - PZMO with very small or 0 target limits: useful—it simply incorporates all z-scores into the metric.
  - PZMO with very large target limits: not useful—PZMO would also be 0, as all z-scores would be ignored.
  - PZMOU: provides PZMO for all "upper" z-scores (i.e. those above upper target limit).
  - PZMOL: provides PZMO for all "lower" z-scores (i.e. those below lower target limit).
- Strengths of PZMO:
  - Capable of reflecting all z-scores (with target size of zero).
  - Reflects dynamic change in the training process.
  - Consistent with existing PZOK approaches.
  - Provision for giving different weights to different types of z-scores.

- Weaknesses of PZMO:
  - PZMO can become large in the presence of artifact, producing feedback when it is not desired. This is because, as the z-scores normalize when the artifact reduces, PZMO "sees" a lot of improvement. But it is improvement from an abnormally noisy situation, and hence is not really to be rewarded. To manage this, designs should include both PZOK and PZMO in the reward mechanism. When artifact is present, PZOK will fall rapidly, thus inhibiting feedback.

PZME (Color Plate 37) provides a measure of the mean size of all z-scores that are outside the target range. For every z-score considered, its distance from zero (normal) is computed, and these are combined into population mean (average). This provides a simple assessment of how abnormal all z-scores are as a group. Different types of z-scores can be given different weight if desired. PZME is intended to be used primarily as an indicator of overall improvement but can also be used for training. Training PZME (downward) would conform the naive principle of simply "training everything toward normal," and is conceptually a step backwards yet is still an important new capability.

The interpretation of PZME is simple. If it has a value of 1.7, for example, then the average size of all the z-scores is simply 1.7. Direction is taken into account so that z-scores above the range are treated the same as z-scores below the target range. There is also a separate function to get the average z-scores in the positive direction and in the negative direction. Technically, PZME is the "mean error" as defined by statistics. In the solar system analogy, PZME is the average distance of all the planets, and hence reflects the overall "size" of the client's z-score solar system. Generally, a smaller solar system is preferable to a larger one.

PZME is intended to be used as an indicator, to see progress within and across sessions. It provides a single number that has a very clear and simple interpretation. It may, for example, be useful in assessing the overall progress, and whether to terminate training. For example, when clients tire, z-scores sometimes are seen to lose their tendency to be improving. If PZME shows an increase for more than three or five minutes, for example, then the client is moving in the wrong direction, and training should be re-evaluated.

PZME also has the potential to be used to create target limits for LZT training. By providing an instantaneous measure of the average length of all z-scores across the board, PZME provides a basis for adjusting target limits for training. While the use of autothresholding is controversial and may or may not be desired in a particular case, PZME provides an objective, sound approach to creating target thresholds that are based on the instantaneous state of the desired z-scores.

For example, the following Event Wizard expression

x = PZOKUL(PZMEU(0), PZMEL(0));

would automatically train PZOK using the average of all positive z-scores as the upper target limit, and the average of all negative z-scores as the lower target limit.

The simplest approach to combining live z-scores would be to add them together (using absolute value) to get a single number. With PZME, we have decided to provide just that; a simple, total assessment of how all the z-scores add up. We leave it to clinical and research progress to determine the utility of PZME for training, control, or for assessment. Intuitively, and from our experience, if trained z-scores are seen to visibly move toward normal, then the PZME variable would also have to go down in a uniform fashion. PZME simply now provides a number that can be used to estimate the total instantaneous condition of all z-scores, treated as a whole.

PZME has the following behavior:

- Minimum value: 0 ("all z-scores are exactly normal").
- Maximum value: unlimited, but typically will not reach as high as 3.0 ("if z-scores are very abnormal").
- Intermediate values: typically 0 to 2.0 ("the average size of all z-scores").
- Limiting behavior:
  - PZME with very small or 0 target limits: useful—it simply incorporates all z-scores into the metric.
  - PZME with very large target limits: not useful—PZME would also be 0, as all z-scores would be ignored.
  - PZMEU: provides PZME for all "upper" z-scores (i.e. those above upper target limit).
  - PZMEL: provides PZME for all "lower" z-scores (i.e. those below lower target limit).
- Strengths of PZME:
  - Extremely simple and intuitive.
  - Capable of reflecting all z-scores (with target size of zero).
  - Reflects total state of the brain.
  - Consistent with existing PZOK approaches.
  - Provision for giving different weights to different types of z-scores.
  - Can be used to develop targets, i.e. autothresholding for LZT.
- Weaknesses of PZME:
  - None yet known.

Color Plate 38 shows live data from actual training, showing PZMO and PZME reflecting the training effects. This shows the effect of changing the target size. The training parameters change in the expected way as the targets are widened.

Z-Bars

The display called Z-Bars shows all z-scores as bars with dynamic lines that show short-term changes. Color Plate 39 shows one such display. This illustrates an important point regarding live z-scores and variability. It can be noted that, among the live z-scores, those with the most variability tend to be the most normal (i.e. a z-score that is averaging near zero is also showing significant variation). Normal z-scores do not stay at zero, but rather move considerably from moment to moment. It is the most deviant z-scores that tend to remain "stuck" and do not vary.

Color Plate 40 shows as many z-scores as are being trained. This panel shows 192 coherence z-scores from 19 channels.

An example of simultaneous text and Z-Bars is shown in Color Plate 41. This demonstrates the ability to pinpoint deviations using the text display, as well as the graphical display.

Z-Maps

Live maps of z-score can be used for training or for following training progress.

"Instantaneous" maps show the moment-to-moment changes, and can change rapidly. "Damped" maps show the damped z-score, which is what is also used in the text display. This provides a more stable map for viewing and biofeedback. Both types of map are useful, depending on the priority. It is possible to display either or both types of map at the same time. Damped z-scores are what are shown in the text and in the colored Z-Bars. Instantaneous z-scores are what are shown by the dynamic lines and dots on the Z-Bars display.

An example of a live Z-Map is shown in Color Plate 42.

Color Plate 43 shows simultaneous Z-Bars and Z-Maps. In this example, low power in delta is evident, and can be seen in the bars as well as the maps.

PZMO is an outgrowth of the PZOK approach, and is an aggregate statistic reflecting change in the outlying z-scores. PZOK tells how many z-scores are within the target range, as a percentage. We usually use a percentage of between 50 percent and 80 percent, which means that a substantial portion of the z-scores are outliers. As a dynamical systems approach, this gives the brain flexibility to "choose" which z-scores to normalize and which to leave as outliers. PZMO is the aggregate momentum of these outliers. It is a measure of their net motion and is a dynamic systems concept. Think of the z-scores as having a life of their own, having mass and velocity. PZMO measures the group momentum and tells you what percentage of the net motion is toward the target range. PZMO is generally below zero, as nothing is moving particularly toward the targets in general. However, when PZMO goes positive, it tells you the net positive movement. A value of 5 percent for PZMO is significant. It means that, in the last instant, there was 5 percent net motion toward the targets. That is a very big deal. This is therefore a "derivative" measure that tells your client that, at that moment, the outliers moved inward. We typically see only a few PZMO reward beeps every few seconds, so it is an added reward. It is like giving the brain a "gold star" when it has particularly good improvement at that moment in time. In my view, it has a similar effect on the brain as the derivatives market had on Wall Street. Small changes can have huge effects, and major learning processes become possible.

PZME is a measure of the mean distance of the outliers from the zero point. It is a measure of the global size of the scattering of outliers in the collection of z-scores. As it moves lower, the outliers are moving closer to the targets. We mostly use this as a long-term statistic throughout the session, watching for a small change, say from 2.5 to 2.2, over the session.

In brief, PZOK only knows the percentage inside the target range; it does not know about the outliers, except that they must be out there someplace. PZMO tells you the net motion of the outliers at any instant. PZME tells you how far out they are in general. While PZMO is a very fast, derivative measure, PZME is a very slow, aggregate measure. It all feeds into a view of the brain and the z-scores as comprising a dynamic system that can determine its own rules for self-regulation if you give it the right information.

Thus, this approach, which we call "Z-Plus," gives you more than one type of information. There are various ways to use PZMO, but one common approach is to give a reward when PZMO rises above zero, indicating net motion toward the targets.

Philosophy of Z-Score Training: Flexibility and Appropriateness versus being "Stuck"

Upon initial consideration, it might seem that z-score-based neurofeedback is based on the concept of making things that are too large small and things that are too small larger. One might also expect that one basic tenet is that everyone should have an "average" EEG. However, upon deeper investigation, it is clear that live z-score neurofeedback is a form of flexibility training. It is evident from Figure 8.18, for example, that the most deviant z-scores (the blue bars) are also those with the least amount of variation (small or no variation lines present). Therefore, the issue is not so much that a particular component is large or small, but that it is stuck.

There are various approaches to live z-score training. The approach used in our laboratory, which was initiated in 2007, has proven to be effective, as well as comprehensive. When we began to do neurofeedback using multiple z-scores, some worried that the information fed back to the trainee would be too complex, and that the brain would be unable to "unravel" all the information. The problem was likened to combing out a ball of knotted string, with no hope for sorting individual strands out. This fear has turned out to be unfounded, and the brain is perfectly suited to interpreting feedback, even if the reward is based upon hundreds, even thousands, of individual z-scores.

9

LORETA NEUROFEEDBACK

There has long been interest and progress in determining the brain activity that underlies the EEG without using invasive sensors. Various solutions to this problem have been developed, and all of them incorporate a solution to the "inverse" problem described previously. As was pointed out, there are an infinite number of possible source configurations that can lead to given measurement, so this has been a difficult problem to solve. Practical solutions require additional assumptions to be made, and may also depend on empirical data, such as actual measurements or trial solutions, in order to limit the possible range of solutions. Generally, the simplest, most likely, or otherwise "best" estimates are what are produced by particular methods. While these approaches have evolved for decades, they have not been relevant to neurofeedback until real-time implementation was possible, allowing calculation and feedback of source information without excessive delay.

Low-resolution electromagnetic tomographic analysis (LORETA) was developed and has been described by Pasqual-Marqui (2002). It is a mathematical technique that uses scalp data from a whole-head EEG and computes an estimate of the cortical electrical activity that could have given rise to that surface potential. Note that this estimate is only one of an infinite number of possible solutions, but it is based upon simplifying principles and has been subjected to independent validation.

sLORETA is based upon the same basic scientific principles as LORETA, but includes three additional important features. The first is that 6,239 voxels are used (the amygdala is not included in sLORETA). The second is that it incorporates an assumption of smoothness into the solution. This determines a unique solution that is intuitively the simplest brain dipole configuration that can lead to the observed surface potentials. The third is that the algorithm has zero localization error.

The introduction of LORETA-based techniques to neurofeedback introduces several important and unique capabilities. It also places certain new demands on the practical aspects of training. The most important and obvious factor introduced by these approaches is that it is possible to provide feedback related to the activity of a particular region, or regions, of the brain, rather than basing training on scalp activity. The ability to train regionally opens the possibility of reinforcing activity in, for example, the anterior cingulated gyrus, or the insula, in contrast to simply Fz or Cz. This has some impact on typical downtraining, such as theta inhibit, in that the feedback will be more directly related to specific activity in the chosen area. Selected brain regions are referred to as "regions of interest" or "ROIs" in practice. More importantly, it is also possible to train particular higher frequencies, such as beta, in a very specific manner. Because of the more localized specificity of higher-frequency activity in the cortex, localized training becomes more important in this regard. It might be harder to justify uptraining beta on Fz, for example, than it would be to do the same training specific to a site known to be exhibiting a deficit, such as the anterior cingulate.

In order to achieve the benefits of localized training, it is necessary to provide sufficient leads to compute the internal "solution." Generally, all 19 10-20 sites are required to do training based on the inverse solution. The solution consists of values computed for thousands of spatial regions, known as "voxels." In the same way that a two-dimensional image can be broken into "pixels," a three-dimensional solid can be broken into these voxels. A key aspect of such localization is the size and number of voxels. LORETA uses approximately 2,300 7-millimeter voxels, while sLORETA and eLORETA use 6,239 5-millimeter voxels.

A second important requirement of practical regionalized training is that the EEG must be free of artifacts. Any contamination in the scalp signals will be included in the computation of the inverse solution. If activity is coming from the eyes or muscles, for example, the assumptions of the computation are violated, and the results will be unreliable.

The LORETA (or sLORETA or eLORETA) computation is based upon a matrix operation that converts the scalp data ("lead field") into the internal brain representation. For example, an sLORETA solution will involve a matrix that has 19 columns and 6,239 rows, and contains three elements in each cell. These elements represent the x, y, and z axes of the dipole solution for each voxel. Therefore, a single solution for one time-point will require $19 \times 6,239 \times 3 = 355623$ computations. At 256 samples per second, and for 10 frequency bands, this equates to over 91 million floating-point computations per second, in addition to the data acquisition, signal processing, and display demands for all 19 channels, plus any images being shown.

Therefore, a significant issue with inverse solutions is the time required for the computation. Traditionally, this has been very long, and complete real-time solutions including graphic displays have not been possible until relatively recently. Solving the problem of delay can be handled in two basic ways. One is to reduce the work by selecting a subset, or representative voxels, for the computation. This approach has been described by Congedo et al. (2004b) and Kaiser (2010). It incorporates assumptions or rationale regarding the specific voxels chosen and their use for feedback. Another approach is to implement the entire mathematical transformation in real time, using specific computer techniques beyond the scope of conventional "programming." Modern personal computer hardware has been increasingly oriented toward the needs of media, animation, and gaming, and graphics hardware has become a sophisticated resource in addition to main computer processing resources. It is possible to exploit the distributed multiprocessing resources designed for these applications in the solution of the inverse calculations, using techniques proprietary to this area. As an example, at the time of writing, a typical sLORETA solution can be computed for all 6,239 voxels at about ½ real time. That means that a 20-second record would take about 40 seconds to compute values for all voxels, for all data points at 256 samples per second. Using advanced media and game-oriented techniques incorporating specialized hardware, it is possible to compute a complete sLORETA solution faster than 10 times real time. For neuro-feedback, it is thus possible to compute inverse solutions for all voxels and all frequency bands in real time and provide immediate feedback for operant training. Using this approach, rather than using a representative voxel for a region, the entire activity of that region can be imaged and fed back. Color Plate 44 shows an example of an sLORETA solution for the cingulate gyrus. The difference in activity from front to back is clearly evident. A single-voxel approach would be limited in its ability to accurately represent the activity of this region because the voxel chosen might not accurately represent the activity of the entire region.

LORETA-based techniques can be combined with z-score concepts to provide assessment and training of voxels based on normative or other references. In order to achieve regionalized z-scores, a reference must be computed for every voxel to be estimated. This increases the size of the reference database considerably, as the typical 19 scalp sites are now replaced by thousands of voxels, and normative data must be known for every voxel.

The voxel data are computed in three dimensions, producing a vector for each voxel. That means that each voxel has not only a magnitude, but also a direction or "moment" associated with it. Theoretically, this dipole will reflect the direction of depolarization of the pyramidal cells in that voxel. Therefore, LORETA-based approaches can be used to estimate voxel activity both as a quantity across time and also as a direction in space.

By combining brain activity images across time, it is possible to visualize and interpret complex sequences of operations, rather than the static representation of a state or condition. For example, the amount of beta activity may be normal in an individual, but the pattern of activation may reveal nuances that only appear in the combined space and time analysis. As one example, Color Plate 45 shows a snapshot of beta activity from a client who was depressed, as well as anxious. While the static QEEG showed no particular abnormality in beta activity, a time review of the animation revealed a pattern of cyclic beta activity between the right dorsolateral frontal cortex, the cingulate gyrus, and the left parietal area. This activation can be interpreted as mediating a negative mood, and alternating rumination that involves the "individual as self." By incorporating this type of information into therapeutic interventions with our without neurofeedback, this dynamic imaging capability provides a valuable illumination of clinically relevant data.

It is possible to combine voxel data into collections that constitute relevant brain regions of interest (ROIs). Examples of these ROIs are shown in the accompanying text box below. When selecting ROIs, the system should compute a suitable representation of the activity of that ROI. The optimal method is to calculate the activity of all of the constituent voxels, and to compute an average or similar metric that adequately represents that region. See Color Plates 46 and 47.

LORETA/sLORETA Regions of Interest (ROIs)

- Frontal lobe
- Limbic lobe
- Occipital lobe
- Parietal lobe
- Sub-lobar
- Temporal lobe
- Angular gyrus
- Anterior cingulate
- Cingulate gyrus
- Cuneus
- Extra-nuclear
- Fusiform gyrus
- Inferior frontal gyrus
- Inferior occipital gyrus
- Inferior parietal lobule
- Inferior temporal gyrus
- Insula
- Lingual gyrus
- Medial frontal gyrus
- Middle frontal gyrus
- Middle occipital gyrus

- Middle temporal gyrus
- Orbital gyrus
- Paracentral lobule
- Parahippocampal gyrus
- Postcentral gyrus
- Posterior cingulate
- Precentral gyrus
- Precuneus
- Rectal gyrus
- Sub-gyral
- Subcallosal gyrus
- Superior frontal gyrus
- Superior occipital gyrus
- Superior parietal lobule
- Superior temporal gyrus
- Supramarginal gyrus
- Transverse temporal gyrus
- Uncus
- Brodman areas 1–11, 13, 17–25, 27–47

10

NEUROFEEDBACK IN PRACTICE

Through practical experience with neurofeedback, practitioners have been able to articulate three principles necessary for effective feedback. In the words of James V. Hardt (1999), it must be "fast," "accurate," and "aesthetic." Another way to capture this would be to say "timely," "correct," and "good" (Sterman, 2008). Essentially, the feedback must provide information in a time frame that will allow temporal binding and learning to occur.

Accuracy means that the signals accurately reflect the brain processes of interest. If the feedback is not accurate, then it can introduce false feedback. In the extreme, spurious reinforcement can lead to confusion, and even superstitious thoughts and behavior (Skinner, 1948).

The feedback must also be aesthetic so that the brain will seek the reward. There must not be undue effort or confusion associated with receiving the reward. If the reward is cryptic or obscure, the brain will not readily adapt to it.

Effective Feedback

- Fast—provides timely information to allow temporal binding.
- Accurate—brain has good information to work with, not ambiguous or superfluous.
- Aesthetic—brain will respond well to the content of the feedback without undue effort or confusion.

Types of Feedback

- Visual
- Auditory
- Vibrotactile
- Real-world devices
- Subliminal/energy feedback

Neurofeedback should be viewed as a means of training self-regulation and achieving normalization, as one component of an overall clinical program. When used in conjunction with other interventions, including cognitive-behavioral and related therapy, lifestyle management, diet and exercise, family dynamic therapy, hypnotherapy, EMDR, or even electrical or magnetic stimulation techniques, it provides a valuable underpinning that can help to potentiate beneficial change. The clinician should be able to understand and anticipate the effects of brain normalization with neural feedback and plan for its use as an element of the overall therapeutic program.

Instructions to the Trainee

- Allow the sounds to come.
- Do not "try" to do anything.
- Allow yourself to learn what it feels like when you get a point.
- Relax and pay attention to the screen.
- Let the sounds tell you when you are in the desired state.

One of the most important factors is the instructions to the trainee. More than one research project has gone astray because a trainee was placed in front of a neural feedback system with no guidance or additional feedback. The process of neural feedback is largely automatic and is certainly not difficult. However, the context and expectations of the trainee must be taken into consideration so that the learning process is facilitated.

It is not surprising that an uninitiated observer might question how neurofeedback could possibly work. There is something mysterious about a child watching a computer monitor and, for some reason, spontaneously getting better. Indeed, neurofeedback may appeal to some who have crystals on the table and seek alternative therapies. Neurofeedback is, in fact, an alternative treatment, but it is moving into the mainstream. More than one parent has certainly watched his or her child staring at a simple game screen and wondered how this could possibly be helping. However, it is a fact that the brain will respond to its environment in an automatic fashion, and that minimal coaching or guidance are needed if the system is well designed and configured. Even a very simple bar graph and tone feedback can be effective in the hands of a knowledgeable clinician.

One of the most common questions from clinicians is "What should I tell the client?" There is little or no published research to guide this decision. However, in experience with clinical art, it has emerged that the simplest and most effective instruction is essentially to "Relax and allow the display or sounds to come." If asked "What should I do?" the response should be "You do nothing." If asked "So I should try to do nothing?" the response is "No, you should not try to do nothing, but you should not try to do anything." Trying to do nothing is not the same as not trying to do something. Allow yourself to learn what it feels like when the feedback comes.

This may seem a somewhat odd topic to discuss in a technical foundations book, but this aspect is critical. Neurofeedback is not a simple treatment that fixes problems. It is a scientifically based technique that can allow the client's brain to learn self-regulation skills. These skills have clinical relevance, and changes in brain regulation will be manifest in symptomatic and subjective changes. It is by defecting these changes that neural feedback has its clinical value. As a clinical tool, neurofeedback should be understood as well as, or better than, any other clinical tool. If a clinician has all the scientific and technical concepts but does not integrate neurofeedback into practice in a clinically sound manner, then the benefits will be limited at best.

Aside from observing the screen and allowing oneself to learn, there is really little else to the experience of neurofeedback. The clinical impact is realized when the trainee begins to experience subjective changes and the clinician then puts these changes into context.

While the intent of the neurofeedback is not to put the trainee under task, it is still possible to allow him or her to engage in other activities while attending to the neural feedback sounds. A partial list of possible activities is shown below. This is also a controversial topic, and some clinicians will insist that neural feedback should either be done with a task or without a task. The reality is that as long as the client is able to relax and be focused, and allow the operant learning to occur, neurofeedback can be effective.

Possible Activities During Neurofeedback

- Reading
- Lego
- Drawing
- Tetris
- Coloring book
- Puzzles
- Homework
- Allow trainee to attain relaxed, focused state even while under a task

---

Neurofeedback Learning Mechanisms

- Classical conditioning
- Concurrent learning
- Habituation
- Self-efficacy
- Generalization
- Transference
- Nonlinear dynamic adaptation

Operant conditioning is the process developed by behaviorists including J. B. Watson (1930) and B. F. Skinner (1956). It depends on an action performed by the organism, and can be basically anything at all. Operant conditioning has been used on cats, mice, pigeons, and flatworms. This type of learning occurs when a reward is paired with some action.

It is not necessary for the trainee to be consciously aware of the properties or changes to himself or herself. There is a naive impression that trainees somehow "learn how to make the brain waves voluntarily, and then do it themselves later on." This is not as accurate a depiction as the recognition that the brain has its own ability to internally self-regulate, and that this self-regulation is largely outside of voluntary, conscious control. There is a famous example of operant conditioning in which a psychology class, as a prank (or as an applied experiment), successfully trained the instructor to stay on one side of the room simply by paying attention to him when he was on the left side and ignoring him when he was on the right side (Sabado, 1970, p. 127). Without any awareness that he was being conditioned, the instructor learned to stay in one particular corner of the room in response to the differential attention provided by the students. According to this account, the professor eventually fell off the left side of the stage. In another version, the students even reversed the experiment later and, simply by shifting their behavior to pay attention when he was on the other side of the room, got him to go there. An online video ("How to condition your professor," www.youtube.com/watch?v=khrjRonCkhw) demonstrates how to use this technique to induce your professor to end the class early. This shows that even a complex behavior can be operantly conditioned without any conscious awareness on the part of the subject. Indeed, this procedure will only work if the professor is not aware of what is happening, as awareness in this example would actually subvert the effect of the conditioning behavior.

The Role of Intention in Neurofeedback

One of the more fascinating, and possibly daunting, aspects of neurofeedback is the role of volition in instrumenting change. There is a tendency in Western society to think of human actions in terms of "voluntary," in the sense that we first create a desire to do something and then instruct our brain to take care of the details. The reality is that this is somewhat backwards. As was seen in our earlier example of the movement-related potential, the brain activity that leads to a voluntary movement precedes the movement by up to 1½ seconds. That means that the very idea of the desire to perform the movement comes *after* that brain activity. As would seem necessary, the very desire to perform the action is a brain event, and hence is the result of brain processes. This challenges the idea that the conscious mind is "in charge" of the brain, and puts the cart on quite the other side of the horse.

What this means to neurofeedback is that the brain is the active agent and that the trainee's conscious awareness is more of a passenger than a pilot, and is certainly not the engine. The driving force for thought and action consists in the dynamic instability of the brain and its proclivity to always seek novelty, fulfillment, stimulation, safety, power, and other goals that it perceives.

Neurofeedback does open the question of causality, particularly with regard to how intentions (mental events) and actions (brain/physical events) are interrelated. The elegant thing here is that neurofeedback does not depend on our understanding or articulation of exactly what is happening. There is a continual feedback loop that involves the brain, its electrical properties, some external hardware, and the client's sensory/perceptual systems, and hence the brain. It is not clear where, or if, the client's conscious awareness is particularly necessary for this process. Indeed, Margaret Ayers (1999) had worked with patients who were comatose, hence not necessarily aware, and got their brains to wake up using an EEG-controlled light held up to their eyes. The further realization that mice and flatworms can be conditioned shows that conscious awareness is not a necessary component of this process.

What is being trained in neurofeedback is simply the brain. The brain in this context can be thought of as a relatively stupid organ that goes about its business by adjusting synapses and transmitters in response to various cues. The brain normally processes an enormous amount of information coming from many directions and does its best to decide what is in its best interests. Note that the brain's best interests are not necessarily the client's best interests. The existence of obsessions, ruminating thoughts, compulsive behavior, and other negative processes bear witness to the fact that the brain can set about doing something that seems to suit some need that it thinks needs to be met, but which does not reflect in the well-being of the client.

A possible subtitle for this book, or at least this chapter, might be "Your Stupid Brain." In this context, neurofeedback is an ideal mechanism for working with and optimizing the stupid brain. Neurofeedback gets involved at a deep, nonverbal level. Neurofeedback does not try to reason with the client or to alter his or her brain activity like a sledge. Rather, neurofeedback provides new information that can open up the brain to options in its own dynamical control. Neurofeedback, in its simplest form, is saying something like "How about less theta for a change?" and allowing the brain to make its own decisions. If the changes result in a new stable state, or one that provides continued benefits to the client, then it will continue to be reinforced after the session is over. If not, the client will not have been harmed and the brain can go back to the way it was.

Figure 10.1 is based upon some of the thinking of the philosopher Jae Guan Kim (1993), relating to a concept called "supervenience." This principle asks whether a change in one domain can possibly happen without a change in another. It does not talk about causality, but about what is possible or not. In our analysis, we recognize that there is a physical brain (denoted "P") that undergoes state changes in time. We suppose that the brain is a physical mechanism obeying the laws of nature so that each state can properly cause the next state. (With quantum uncertainty, we still assign sequential states to the system, even if they are not entirely deterministic.) Kim states that the mind supervenes on the brain, which is to say that if two brain states are identical, then the associated mental states are also identical. This means that while there may be many brain states that produce a given mental state (e.g. many ways to worry), once a brain state is specified, the mental state that it produces is determined.

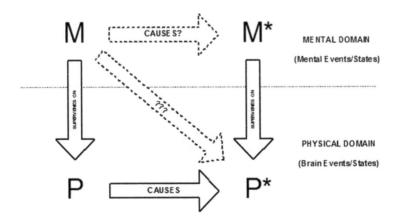

Figure 10.1 The supervenience relationship helps to define the connection between brain and mind in terms of causal paths.

If neurofeedback is to make sense, it needs to make sense in this context. What arises is whether the mental realm really has any autonomy or if it is merely an alternate representation of the brain. It is interesting to note that while talk therapy "thinks" it is operating on the realm of the mental, pharmacotherapy "thinks" that it is operating on the realm of the physical. The fact that we so readily go from one to the other in mental health treatment attests to the fact that there is an implicit assumption that these are two ways of looking at the same thing.

Neurofeedback, therefore, while it appears to operate on the level of the client watching a screen or hearing sounds, and "knowing" that something is happening, may operate at an entirely different level. In the same way that the professor found himself on one side or the other of the room, the brain finds itself in various configurations, which are either reinforced or not, depending on a complex set of criteria. Neurofeedback introduces entirely new criteria that have not been part of human experience for all of the millennia of our existence. Within the past several decades, this door has opened, and now provides a new paradigm for assessment and change. While it is biologically based, it is not fatalistic and does not pigeonhole clients into diagnoses, or even into symptoms. It looks for dysfunction at the level of self-regulation and introduces mechanisms of change that have no precedent in mental health care, with the possible exception of Thomas Edison's brass ball and pie plate (Henslin, 2009).

11

SESSION MANAGEMENT
AND CONTROL

It is useful at this point to ask the fundamental question "What is the purpose of neurofeedback?" It may appear that its purpose is to alleviate some disorder or to change some particular brain rhythm or connection. At the lowest level, the purpose of neurofeedback is to produce an artificially constructed reality that will affect the choices made by the brain in relation to its own self-regulation. The key to neurofeedback is to present the brain with information that is related to its own function and that will facilitate beneficial change. The basic mechanism for this change is presenting information that is "differential," which means that it serves to differentiate one thing from another. In the purest sense, a feedback tone or video serve only to mark moments in time and to tell the brain whether to label certain time intervals in a positive or neutral fashion. The mechanism of neuro-feedback relies on distinguishing one moment in time from another, and allowing the brain to decide what to do with that information.

In a simple example, if a reward is presented when theta is below some threshold, then the brain will learn to differentiate that state. If it is a beneficial state, and the brain can achieve better balance or focus, then that state change may become learned for future use. However, the key element of the feedback is its contingency, which is to say it is contingent on some condition. As is true with all learning paradigms, the choice of what makes the reward forthcoming is the crux of the value of the training.

Goals of Neurofeedback

- Improve self-regulation.
- Achieve flexible and appropriate brain states.
- Normalize connectivity.
- Address functionality, not symptoms.
- Provide lasting change.

Protocol Selection and Design

In planning a neurofeedback session, the protocol must be defined. This can be as simple as "reduce theta at this location" or as complex as "train coherence between these two sites up while reducing beta in another location." In current technology, it is possible to design protocols such as "normalize connectivity across the rear of the head in the alpha and beta bands while keeping theta and high beta at minimal levels." All of these protocols define some underlying brain dynamic that will have clinical relevance as it is achieved through operant training.

Whenever using a protocol that appeals to the notions of "larger," "smaller," or "within normal ranges," the concept of a threshold arises. Theresholds are the decision points, and every protocol, no matter how simple or how complicated, appeals to the notion of some type of threshold. The threshold defines the contingency, in that it tells the system when, based upon the EEG parameters, the rewards will be forthcoming and when they will not.

The use of thresholding is one of the most important and also controversial topics in neurofeedback. A threshold consists of a value that is used as a decision point in creating feedback. Thresholds can be set by the manual methods, automatic methods, or a combination of both.

Thresholding

- Sets amplitude criterion for rewards.
- Compares signal amplitude with set value.
- Can be constant, or can be varying.
- Percent time over threshold is indicator of how often signal exceeds threshold.

Thresholding Facts

- Threshold is generally amplitude value but can be any metric.
- Feedback is controlled via thresholds for each trained component.
- Component may be "enhance" ("go") or "inhibit" ("stop").
- May use more than one component in combination in a protocol.
- "Percent time over threshold" (percent TOT) is average time the component is above threshold.

Targets are generally one of two types. Enhanced, reinforced, or "uptrained" targets are conditions that lead to the possibility of reward. Inhibit or "downtrained" targets remove the possibility of reinforcement. By using combinations of reinforcements and inhibits, the training can be configured to lead the trainee toward any desired state, or even combination of states. The protocol can be described in terms of the percentage of time that enhance or inhibit conditions are met. The total rate of reinforcement will be the mathematic combination of all of these conditions, which translates into the overall success rate of the training protocol.

Threshold Targets

- Enhance—being over threshold allows positive feedback:
  - reward rate = percent TOT.
- Inhibit—being over threshold inhibits feedback:
  - success is being below threshold;
  - reward rate would be 100 − percent TOT.
- Total reward rate is product of individual success rates for each component.

The following examples serve to illustrate the importance and value of adjusting thresholds based upon the relevant contingency to be emphasized for operant learning. A critical aspect of learning is that the individual will discern precisely when rewards are forthcoming and reinforce that state. As in the previously described example of the college professor, an organism does not have to be consciously aware of the learning process. Whatever state or condition is rewarded will tend to be reinforced. Thus, the time-specificity of feedback is translated into state-specificity of the learned behavior.

In the first example, which is a typical set of threshold settings, there is one enhance and two inhibits. As is typical, this example uses a low inhibit, such as delta or theta, a midrange enhance, such as alpha, low beta, or beta, and a high inhibit, such as high beta. If the enhance band is set to reinforce 60 percent of the time, and the low inhibit is true 20 percent of the time, and the high inhibit is true 10 percent of the time, then the total success rate will be 43 percent. In this case, the inhibits are in effect relatively infrequently so that the main differential that the trainee will be exposed to is the presence of the midrange enhance. This, therefore, becomes emphasized in the training.

Threshold Example 1

- Low inhibit (theta)—20 percent TOT:
  - 80 percent success rate = 100 − 20
- Midrange enhance (SMR)—60 percent TOT:
  - 60 percent success rate
- High inhibit (high beta)—10 percent TOT:
  - 90 percent success rate = 100 − 90
- Expected reward rate:
  - $0.8 \times 0.6 \times 0.9 = 0.43 = 43$ percent
- Midrange enhance is emphasized

In the second example, the target thresholds are changed so that the contingencies are now 80 percent enhance, 40 percent on the low inhibit, and 10 percent on the high inhibit. As shown, the total reward contingency is still 43 percent. However, the client is now receiving more information relative to the low inhibit because the midrange enhance is now significantly "easier." The training experience will weighted more toward discerning the absence of theta, and less toward the production of SMR. This would be a useful strategy to use with a beginning child, for example, whose first task would be to learn to reduce theta, before the production of SMR becomes a the focus of training.

Threshold Example 2

- Theta inhibit—40 percent TOT
- SMR enhance—80 percent TOT
- High beta inhibit—10 percent TOT
- Expected reward rate:
  - $0.6 \times 0.8 \times 0.9 = 0.43 = 43$ percent
- Theta inhibit is emphasized

In this final example, the thresholds are further adjusted so that the enhance band is above threshold 100 percent of the time. The net result of this maneuver is to essentially ignore this band. It is thus removed from the training experience. Rather, the theta inhibit is set for 60 percent time above threshold, and the high inhibit is set to never be above threshold.

The total reinforcement rate is still 43 percent. However, the training experience is now entirely that of theta inhibition.

Threshold Example 3

- Theta inhibit—57 percent TOT
- SMR enhance—100 percent TOT
- High beta inhibit—0 percent TOT
- Expected reward rate:
  - $0.43 \times 1.0 \times 1.0 = 0.40 = 43$ percent
- Theta inhibit is all there is—theta "squash"

These examples serve to illustrate how neurofeedback can be configured so as to "titrate" the balance of training conditions. In a manner analogous to the use of combinations of medications in approaching medical treatment, neurofeedback can be configured specifically to target particular brain states and operant behaviors. In this manner, even though the underlying mechanism is quite simple, that of modulation of the concentration/ relaxation cycle in the brain, the configuration of the neurofeedback protocol introduces significant target specificity that can be used to reinforce particular brain states, and even locations, via selective feedback.

In the same way that these adjustments lead to specificity in time, they can also lead to specificity in space. For example, if the system is configured to only reinforce alpha at a particular location, such as the back of the head, then the client will learn to produce alpha in that location. The ability to select location is not unlike that of a strobe light, which is a light that turns on at particular times to reveal a moving object only at specific times. A strobe light can be used to "stop" a moving wheel by flashing only when the wheel is in a particular position. Similarly, if the neurofeedback protocol is configured to reinforce only a particular location and condition, then the brain will learn to reinforce that condition. When used in conjunction with advanced localization techniques such as LORETA or sLORETA, neurofeedback can produce very specific training effects, which are reflected in localization in space, as well as in time.

It is important to recognize the role of the inhibit bands in ensuring that the reinforced overall state is appropriate. In early EEG biofeedback devices, only the reinforced band was monitored. Typically, the individual was rewarded whenever signals in a filter set to the alpha frequency band exceeded a threshold level. A significant concern arose, in that if the trainee did anything to raise this level, including blinking eyes, moving, or creating muscle tension, then a reward would be forthcoming. This made it possible to reinforce these actions, as well as actual alpha activity. Until inhibit bands, also known as "guard" bands, were introduced, this problem could not be overcome and results of "alpha" training were inconsistent.

Another strategy is to use relative power rather than absolute values in determining feedback. In this case, there is an automatic inhibition of signals outside the target band. Another way to look at relative power is as "percent energy" for a band. For example, if the percentage of alpha is rewarded whenever it exceeds 40 percent, then the client will experience rewards when his or her alpha becomes 40 percent or more of the power. One advantage of this simple approach is that, if the client produces out-of-band energy, such as eye blinks or muscle tension, this will tend to reduce the percentage of alpha accordingly. Therefore, the client will not receive rewards when these confounding signals are present, and the effect will be to inhibit any out-of-band activity without the need for explicit inhibits on these frequency ranges.

The question inevitably arises of when and how to adjust thresholds. This question is as old as operant training itself, and has fundamental importance. Unfortunately (or fortunately), there is no simple answer. This question is as complicated as the entire topic of learning, and any method that introduces contingency is a feasible approach. As it turns out, a wide range of philosophies and practices are in use, and will likely continue into the foreseeable future. This reflects the art of neurofeedback and the importance of individual differences between clinicians, as well as between clients.

Because neurofeedback is based upon the trainee's experience, it has elements of art and science. This is particularly relevant when determining the strategy used to set thresholds, as these decisions effectively shape this experience. While certain fundamental rules of operant learning are at play, there is still flexibility in particular decisions, and these will depend to some extent on the preferences of the clinician, as well as the client, and the particular goals. The possible strategies and their considerations are summarized in the text box below. To summarize briefly, it is possible to justify the adjustment of thresholds from one extreme, which is to fix them without change throughout a training program, to the other extreme, which is to adjust them continually.

If thresholds are set once at the beginning of training, and never adjusted, there is the benefit that the trainee will see the effects of his or her improvement over time and be rewarded for progress. One disadvantage is that the training may become too easy over time because the targets are not adjusted in response to improvement in performance. One solution to this is to move to the next level, which is to adjust them once for each session. In this case, the client can be told of the threshold changes, such as "Today, we will use a target of six and see how you do." It would be important in this case to tell the trainee where the thresholds are set each day as part of the reward process. Some practitioners, however, want to emphasize the use of an "optimal" rate of reward, and adjust thresholds every few minutes. In this case, the feedback can also include a periodic display of the progress in terms of the component values themselves so that the trainee can see his or her own progress. Finally, some practitioners will arrange for thresholds to be adjusted continually so that the client is informed whenever the signals go "above where they have been recently," arguing that this will reward any improvement, even over short periods of time.

When to Adjust Thresholds?

- Never:
  – Do not frustrate trainee.
  – Allow to see improvement in scores.
- Once for each session:
  – Tell trainee new threshold.
  – Goal of consistent number of points per session.
- Every 2–5 minutes:
  – Optimal rate of reward.
  – Show trainee improvement in EEG scores.
- Continually:
  – Brain is a dynamical system.
  – Provide information regarding emergent variability.

Clearly, both extremes of this decision process have disadvantages, which are reduced in the middle ground. Therefore, adjusting thresholds for a particular session, or possibly readjusting them periodically, tends to be more common. It should also be noted that threshold adjustment, particularly when it is done automatically ("autothresholding") is controversial, and some practitioners are strongly against this practice. It can be argued that if thresholds are changed too often, then the trainee is training the biofeedback system, not the other way around.

Sessions can be continuous, lasting for 10, 20, or more minutes, or they can be broken into "trials" or "runs." These are often separated by brief pauses or breaks. These are, again, individual decisions that will depend on the training and experience of the clinician, as well as the particulars of the task. For example, alpha training for deep relaxation is often conducted in a single, continuous session, facilitating the achievement of the relaxed, internalized state. SMR or beta training, on the other hand, tend to have a "task" aspect, and can be punctuated by periodic pauses every two, three, or five minutes, during which the trainee rests and reviews session progress.

Another consideration in neurofeedback is how many sessions to use and how long sessions should last. These are, again, very individual decisions based upon a variety of factors. Such issues as seriousness of the problem, availability of the trainee, and travel issues may come into play. As a general rule, neurofeedback will be done no less than once a week so that learned gains can be reinforced and retained. At the other extreme, training more than once or twice a day, day after day, represents an extreme. This can be used if a client has to travel a long distance for neurofeedback and is coming in for an intensive treatment program. In cases of difficulty reaching the clinician, one option is to consider home training, but only after several in-office sessions and appropriate training of the parents or other family members who will be assisting the client.

Sessions generally last less than an hour, with the exception of when alpha/theta training is used to achieve deep states, and is used in conjunction with psychotherapy, guided imagery, or related interventions. It is typical for the duration of actual neurofeedback training to last for a minimum of about 10 minutes, and a maximum of about 30 minutes, in most clinical applications. It is often possible to determine the optimal session length by monitoring the progress of the relevant EEG variables, as well as the client's subjective report. In particular, if the EEG values start to deviate, indicating fatigue or loss of connection to the learning goals, or if the client reports that he or she is getting tired or bored, training should be discontinued for that session.

The number of sessions used will vary. Some clients may report results in less than 5 or 10 sessions, and wish to move onto other therapies or consider their treatment done. Others may require 40 or more sessions, depending on the severity and permanence of their condition. When neurofeedback is used in pervasive conditions such as autism spectrum disorder (ASD), continued neurofeedback may be indicated, with the number of sessions reaching or exceeding 100.

12

MINI-Q ASSESSMENT AND TRAINING METHODS

The MINI-Q is an approach to assessment that bridges the gap between single-channel EEG and the use of a full-head EEG. In its simplest form, a single channel of EEG is recorded for a short period of time, then the sensor is moved to another location, and the process is repeated. It is practical to use this procedure for a short time, up to about 10 minutes, and obtain useful results. If the process takes much longer, changes in alertness or drowsiness can cause results to be inconsistent. As one approach to minimize this concern, it is also possible to use a two-channel or four-channel EEG and acquire the channels in combinations. For example, by taking successive one-minute samples with a two-channel EEG, it is possible to acquire 12 channels in six minutes, which represents a useful set of compromises.

When performing a MINI-Q with two or four channels, it is significantly more convenient to use a device that performs the channel changing, or "switching," automatically. Some system providers offer such devices, along with software that provides additional conveniences, such as timing the session, prompting the operator, and arranging the data for ease of analysis. It is possible to acquire reasonably useful amplitude data and even topographic maps using the MINI-Q approach. For example, using a four-channel EEG, it is possible to acquire 20 channels of data in five minutes, thus acquiring every one of the 10-20 channels. It is possible, in addition, to measure the connectivity between any pairs of sensors that are acquired simultaneously.

Figure 12.1 shows a typical EEG tracing from a MINI-Q assessment. The successive traces are shown "stacked" so that the entire set of sensor channels can be seen on the recording. It is important to note that channels that are not acquired simultaneously can still be displayed together, so that features that appear at the same horizontal location may not have occurred at the same time. This makes it impossible to read the EEG field potentials that are visible when a full whole-head EEG is taken. This loss of simultaneous data acquisition is one of the major disadvantages of the MINI-Q method. Figure 12.2 shows a typical spreadsheet representation of the data

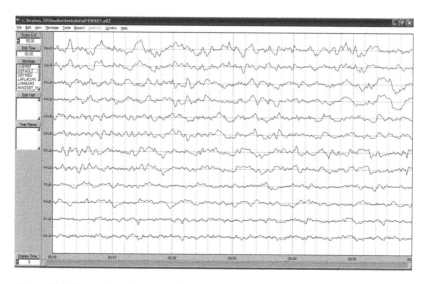

Figure 12.1 Typical EEG tracings from a MINI-Q recording.

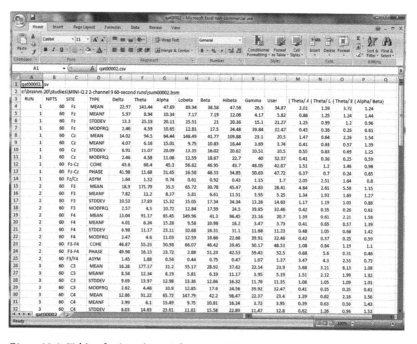

Figure 12.2 Table of values derived from a MINI-Q assessment and analysis.

computed by the software. This permits rapid visual inspection of salient results. Examples of the key attributes that can be seen in a MINI-Q include general amplitude levels of key component, amount of front-back and left-right asymmetry, presence of EEG abnormalities, and peak alpha frequency.

Attributes Measurable via MINI-Q

- General levels of theta, alpha, beta, etc.
- Relative amounts of alpha front to back.
- Relative amounts of beta front to back.
- Asymmetry in frontal alpha.
- Peak alpha frequency, front and back.
- Presence of visually evident abnormalities.
- Visualization of excess slow activity.
- Visualization of excess fast activity.

Functional Analysis of Four-Channel Sensor Positions and Use with Live Z-Scores

A Window to Four-Channel EEG Assessment and Training

In addition to being useful as an assessment method, the MINI-Q approach also provides a capability for efficient training of brain locations, as well as functional "hubs." By combining sites related to particular functions, the MINI-Q approach provides the ability to target particular sets of brain functions for neurofeedback. In these examples, the MINI-Q is used to provide eight positions, each selecting four channels. With a rear push button, a ninth position is available. The sensors for the positions are shown below.

Position	Active 1	Active 2	Active 3	Active 4
1	Fz	Cz	T3	T4
2	F3	F4	O1	O2
3	C3	C4	F7	F8
4	P3	P4	T5	T6
5	Fp1	Fp2	Pz	Oz (not 10-20)
5a	T3	T4	Pz	Oz (not 10-20)
6	O1	O2	C3	C4
7	F7	F8	F3	F4
8	T5	T6	Fz	Cz

In each position, the MINI-Q II provides four sites and six connection paths between them. By using particular MINI-Q II positions for training, it is possible to target specific brain functions in an efficient manner and train all four sites. When used with live z-score training capability, it is possible to train all four sites, in addition to their six interconnections. This provides an efficient means to target specific functions. When used with four channels, the live z-score software provides 248 training variables as z-scores:

- For each channel, for each of eight bands: absolute and relative power (4 × 16 = 64 z-scores).
- For each channel: 10 power ratios (4 × 10 = 40 z-scores).
- For each pair of channels (six pairs): coherence, phase, asymmetry (6 × 24 = 144 z-scores).

The following pages detail the brain locations and functions accessed by each MINI-Q II position. The functional interpretations are based on Walker et al. (2007). Each position provides a "window" into the trainee's brain, with unique capabilities for assessment and training. By referring to these charts, along with the live z-scores, it becomes possible to monitor and train specific brain functions using four channels in a convenient and optimal manner.

Based upon the following detailed explanations, each of the nine possible MINI-Q II settings becomes a "window" into particular aspects of brain function. When the brain is analyzed by taking sets of four channels in particular patterns, each pattern demonstrates a particular set of brain functional elements and their interactions.

For purposes of general understanding, it is possible to classify each MINI-Q II position in terms of the brain activities that it reflects, and how these are integrated into the overall function of the brain. In addition, by considering the effects of hypo-coherence or hyper-coherence in each possible pair, it is possible to address modular interactions and place them in the context of clinical signs.

Each of the positions is described in detail on the following pages. For a summary account of their properties, the following nomenclature can emerge. For the benefit of succinctness, each position is further identified with an overall role, and a role "image" of that brain subsystem, the role that it subserves. It is anticipated that this interpretation will be of value in clinical assessment, and management of trainees, in cases in which particular functional subsystems can be identified for purposes of optimizing clinical outcomes.

Position	Brain site(s)	Functional aspects	Overall role
1	Frontal; Temporal	Remembering and planning	Goalsetting; "Captain"
2	Frontal; Occipital	Seeing and planning	Lookout; "Guide"
3	Central; Frontal	Doing and expressing	Outward Expression; "Actor"
4	Parietal; Temporal	Perceiving and understanding	Interpreting the world; "Scholar"
5	Prefrontal; Parietal	Attending and perceiving	Observer; "Owl"
5a	Temporal; Parietal	Remembering and perceiving	Ponderer; "Sage"
6	Occipital; Central	seeing and acting	Outward actions; "Hero"
7	Frontal	Planning and expressing	Planner; "Oracle"
8	Temporal; Frontocentral	Understanding and doing	Skilled; "Adept"

It is evident that, based upon this arrangement, this method provides a useful way to separate out functional subsystems in the brain, and to assess and train them in a systematic manner using four channels of EEG. Depending on the outcome of the entire MINI-Q (or QEEG) analysis, it becomes possible to define the functional aspects that are addressed by each of the possible MINI-Q II positions, and to design training protocols around them.

In addition to being used to normalize brain function based on z-scores, this method can also be used for peak performance or mental fitness applications, such as alpha synchrony, coherence training, activation ("squash") training, or disruptive training, such as bi-hemispheric. These areas can be further pursued using this method to design protocols that optimize brain function in specified subsystems toward specific goals. It is also possible to design four-channel training protocols based on QEEG results or specific training goals.

MINI-Q II Position 1

"Remembering and Planning"

Summary: This position provides a primary window to motor planning of the lower extremities, sensorimotor integration, and logical and emotional memory formation and storage. Secondary functions include phonological processing, hearing, and ambulation.

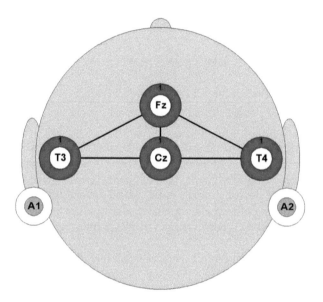

Figure 12.3 Sites: Fz Cz T3 T4 "Frontal Midline and Temporal Lobes."

10-20 territory modules	Principal function	Other functions
Fz	Motor planning of both lower extremities (BLE) and midline	Running, walking, kicking
Cz	Sensorimotor integration both lower extremities (BLE) and midline	Ambulation
T3	Logical (verbal) memory formation and storage	Phonological processing, hearing (bilateral) suppression of tinnitus
T4	Emotional (non-verbal memory formation and storage)	Hearing (bilateral), suppression of tinnitus, autobiographical memory storage

Coherence	Result of hypo-coherence	Result of hyper-coherence
Fz-Cz	Less efficient midline motor action/ midline sensorimotor integration	Lack of flexibility of midline motor action/midline sensorimotor integration
Fz-T3	Less efficient logical memory/ midline motor actions	Lack of flexibility of logical memory/ midline motor actions
Fz-T4	Less efficient emotional memory/ midline motor actions	Lack of flexibility of emotional memory/midline motor actions
Cz-T3	Less efficient logical memory/ midline sensorimotor integration	Lack of flexibility of logical memory/ midline sensorimotor integration
Cz-T4	Less efficient emotional memory/ midline sensorimotor integration	Lack of flexibility of emotional memory/midline sensorimotor integration
T3-T4	Less efficient logical memory/ emotional memory	Lack of flexibility of logical memory/ emotional memory

Source: Based on Walker et al. (2007)

MINI-Q II Position 2

"Seeing and Planning"

Summary: This position provides a primary window to motor planning of the upper extremities, motor actions, and visual processing. Secondary functions include fine motor coordination, mood elevation, pattern recognition, and visual sensations and perception.

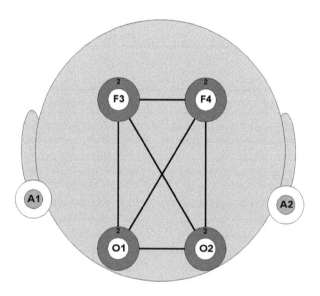

Figure 12.4 Sites: F3 F4 O1 O2 "Frontal and Occipital Homologous Sites."

10-20 territory modules	Principal function	Other functions
F3	Motor planning right upper extremity (RUE)	Fine motor coordination, mood elevation
F4	Motor planning left upper extremity (LUE)	Fine motor coordination (left hand)
O1	Visual processing right half of space	Pattern recognition, color perception, movement perception, black/white perception, edge perception
O2	Visual processing left half of space	Pattern recognition, color perception, movement perception, black/white perception, edge perception

Coherence	Result of hypo-coherence	Result of hyper-coherence
F3-F4	Less efficient motor actions RUE/ motor actions LUE	Lack of flexibility motor actions RUE/motor actions LUE
F3-O1	Less efficient motor actions RUE/ visual sensations R	Lack of flexibility of logical memory/ midline motor actions
F3-O2	Less efficient motor actions RUE/ visual sensations L	Lack of flexibility of emotional memory/midline motor actions
F4-O1	Less efficient motor actions LUE/ visual sensations R	Lack of flexibility of motor actions LUE/visual sensations R
F4-O2	Less efficient motor actions LUE/ visual sensations L	Lack of flexibility of motor actions LUE/visual sensations L
O1-O2	Less efficient visual sensations R/ visual sensations L	Lack of flexibility of visual sensations L/visual sensations R

Source: Based on Walker et al. (2007)

MINI-Q II Position 3

"Doing and Expressing"

Summary: This position provides a primary window to sensorimotor integration, and verbal and emotional expression, motor actions of the upper extremities, visual sensations, verbal/sensorimotor integration, and verbal/ emotional expression. Secondary functions include alerting and calming responses, handwriting, drawing, and mood regulation.

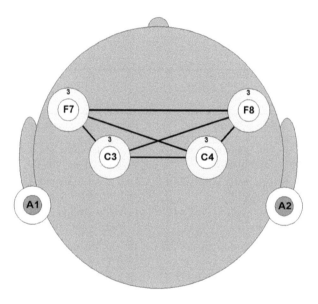

Figure 12.5 Sites: C3 C4 F7 F8 "Mesial Motor Strip and Lateral Frontal Homologous Sites."

10-20 territory modules	Principal function	Other functions
C3	Sensorimotor integration right upper extremity (RUE)	Alerting responses Handwriting (right hand)
C4	Sensorimotor integration left upper extremity (LUE)	Calming Handwriting (left hand)
F7	Verbal expression	Speech fluency Mood regulation (cognitive)
F8	Emotional expression	Drawing (right hand) Mood regulation (endogenous)

Coherence	Result of hypo-coherence	Result of hyper-coherence
C3-C4	Less efficient sensorimotor integration RUE/sensorimotor integration	Lack of flexibility of sensorimotor integration RUE/sensorimotor integration
C3-F7	Less efficient verbal/sensorimotor integration RUE	Lack of flexibility of verbal/sensorimotor integration RUE
C3-F8	Less efficient emotional expression/sensorimotor integration RUE	Lack of flexibility of emotional expression/sensorimotor integration RUE
C4-F7	Less efficient emotional expression/sensorimotor integration LUE	Lack of flexibility of emotional expression/sensorimotor integration LUE
C4-F8	Less efficient emotional expression/sensorimotor integration LUE	Lack of flexibility of emotional expression/sensorimotor integration LUE
F7-F8	Less efficient verbal/emotional expression	Lack of flexibility of verbal/emotional expression

Source: Based on Walker et al. (2007)

MINI-Q II Position 4

"Perceiving and Understanding"

Summary: This position provides a primary window to perception and cognitive processing, spatial relations, and logical and emotional understanding, memory, and perceptions. Secondary functions include spatial relations sensations, calculations, multimodal interactions, recognition of words and faces, and auditory processing.

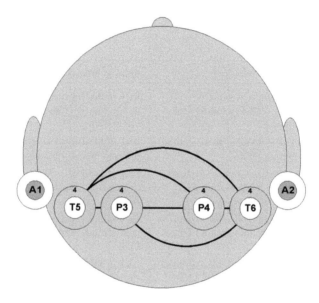

Figure 12.6 Sites: P3 P4 T5 T6 "Parietal and Posterior Temporal Homologous Sites."

10-20 territory modules	Principal function	Other functions
P3	Perception (cognitive processing) right half of space	Spatial relations Sensations Multimodal sensations Calculations Praxis Reasoning (verbal)
P4	Perception (cognitive processing) left half of space	Spatial relations Multimodal interactions Praxis Reasoning (nonverbal)
T5	Logical (verbal) understanding	Word recognition Auditory processing
T6	Emotional understanding	Facial recognition Symbol recognition Auditory processing

Coherence	Result of hypo-coherence	Result of hyper-coherence
P3-P4	Less efficient perceptions R/ perceptions L	Lack of flexibility of perceptions R/ perceptions L
P3-T5	Less efficient logical memory/ perception R	Lack of flexibility of logical memory/ perception R
P3-T6	Less efficient emotional memory/ perceptions R	Lack of flexibility of emotional memory/perceptions R
P4-T5	Less efficient logical memory/ perceptions L	Lack of flexibility of logical memory/ perception L
P4-T6	Less efficient emotional memory/ perceptions L	Lack of flexibility of emotional memory/perceptions L
T5-T6	Less efficient logical memory/ emotional memory	Lack of flexibility of logical memory/ emotional memory

Source: Based on Walker et al. (2007)

MINI-Q II Position 5

"Attending and Perceiving"

Summary: This position provides a primary window to logical and emotional attention, perception, and visual processing. Secondary functions include planning, decision-making, task completion, sense of self, self-control, and route finding.

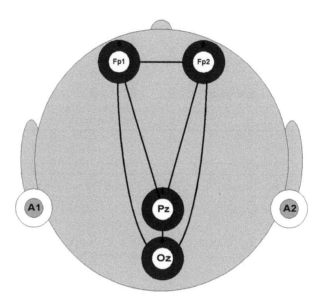

Figure 12.7 Sites: Fp1 Fp2 Pz Oz "Prefrontal Homologous and Posterior Midline Sites."

10-20 territory modules	Principal function	Other functions
Fp1	Logical attention	Orchestrate network interactions planning Decision-making Task completion Working memory
Fp2	Emotional attention	Judgment Sense of self Self-control Restraint of impulses
Pz	Perception midline	Spatial relations Praxis Route finding
Oz (not a 10-20 position)	Visual processing of space	Primary visual sensation

Coherence	Result of hypo-coherence	Result of hyper-coherence
Fp1-Fp2	Less efficient integration of logical/ emotional attention	Lack of flexibility of integrating logical/emotional attention
Fp1-Pz	Logical attention/midline perception	Lack of flexibility of logical attention/midline perception
Fp1-Oz	(no data)	(no data)
Fp2-Pz	Less efficient emotional attention/ midline perception	Lack of flexibility of emotional attention/midline perception
Fp2-Oz	(no data)	(no data)
Pz-Oz	(no data)	(no data)

Source: Based on Walker et al. (2007)

MINI-Q II Position 5a (Rear Push Button OUT)

"Remembering and Perceiving"

Summary: This position provides a primary window to logical and emotional memory formation and storage, perception, and visual processing. Secondary functions include phonological processing, hearing, spatial relations, and visual sensation.

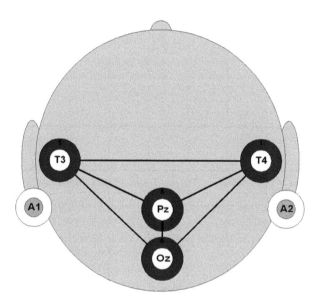

Figure 12.8 Sites: T3 T4 Pz Oz "Temporal Lobes and Posterior Midline."

10-20 territory modules	Principal function	Other functions
T3	Logical (verbal) memory formation and storage	Phonological processing, hearing (bilateral) suppression of tinnitus
T4	Emotional (nonverbal memory formation and storage	Hearing (bilateral), suppression of tinnitus, autobiographical memory storage
Pz	Perception midline	Spatial relations Praxis Route finding
Oz (not a 10-20 position)	Visual processing of space	Primary visual sensation

Coherence	Result of hypo-coherence	Result of hyper-coherence
T3-T4	Less efficient logical memory/ emotional memory	Lack of flexibility of logical memory/ emotional memory
T3-Pz	Less efficient logical memory/ midline perception	Lack of flexibility of logical memory/ midline perception
T3-Oz	(no data)	(no data)
T4-Pz	Less efficient logical memory/ midline perception	Lack of flexibility of logical memory/ midline perception
T4-Oz	(no data)	(no data)
Pz-Oz	(no data)	(no data)

Source: Based on Walker et al. (2007)

MINI-Q II Position 6

"Seeing and Acting"

Summary: This position provides a primary window to visual sensory processing, and sensorimotor integration of the upper extremities. Secondary functions include pattern recognition, perception of color, movement, black/white, edges, alerting and calming responses, handwriting, and logical and emotional memory and perception.

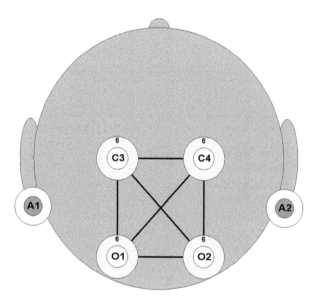

Figure 12.9 Sites: O1 O2 C3 C4 "Occipital and Motor Strip Homologous Sites."

10-20 territory modules	Principal function	Other functions
O1	Visual processing right half of space	Pattern recognition, color perception, movement perception, black/white perception, edge perception
O2	Visual processing left half of space	Pattern recognition, color perception, movement perception, black/white perception, edge perception
C3	Sensorimotor integration right upper extremity (RUE)	Alerting responses Handwriting (right hand)
C4	Sensorimotor integration left upper extremity (LUE)	Calming Handwriting (left hand)

Coherence	Result of hypo-coherence	Result of hyper-coherence
O1-O2	Less efficient visual sensations R/visual sensations L	Lack of flexibility of visual sensations L/visual sensations R
O1-C3	Less efficient sensorimotor integration RUE/visual sensations R	Lack of flexibility of sensorimotor integration RUE/visual sensations R
O1-C4	Less efficient sensorimotor integration LUE/visual sensations	Lack of flexibility of sensorimotor integration LUE/visual sensations
O2-C3	Less efficient sensorimotor integration RUE/visual sensations L	Lack of flexibility of sensorimotor integration RUE/visual sensations L
O2-C4	Less efficient sensorimotor integration LUE/visual sensations	Lack of flexibility of sensorimotor integration LUE/visual sensations
C3-C4	Less efficient sensorimotor integration RUE/sensorimotor integration L	Lack of flexibility of sensorimotor integration RUE/sensorimotor integration L

Source: Based on Walker et al. (2007)

MINI-Q II Position 7

"Planning and Expressing"

Summary: This position provides a primary window to verbal and emotional expression, motor planning of the upper extremities, and motor actions. Secondary functions include speech fluency, mood regulation, and fine motor coordination.

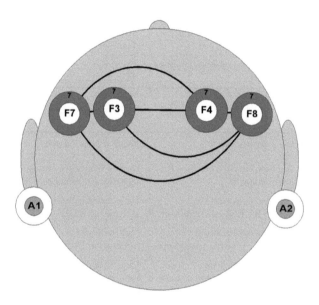

Figure 12.10 Sites: F7 F8 F3 F4 "Full Frontal Lobes Homologous Sites."

10-20 territory modules	Principal function	Other functions
F7	Verbal expression	Speech fluency Mood regulation (cognitive)
F8	Emotional expression	Drawing (right hand) Mood regulation (endogenous)
F3	Motor planning right upper extremity (RUE)	Fine motor coordination, mood elevation
F4	Motor planning left upper extremity (LUE)	Fine motor coordination (left hand)

Coherence	Result of hypo-coherence	Result of hyper-coherence
F7-F8	Less efficient verbal/emotional expression	Lack of flexibility of verbal/emotional expression
F7-F3	Less efficient verbal/motor actions R	Lack of flexibility of verbal/motor actions R
F7-F4	Less efficient verbal/motor actions L	Lack of flexibility of verbal/motor actions L
F8-F3	Less emotional expression/motor actions RUE	Lack of flexibility of emotional expression/motor actions RUE
F8-F4	Less emotional expression/motor actions LUE	Lack of flexibility of emotional expression/motor actions LUE
F3-F4	Less efficient motor actions RUE/motor actions LUE	Lack of flexibility motor actions RUE/motor actions LUE

Source: Based on Walker et al. (2007)

MINI-Q II Position 8

"Understanding and Doing"

Summary: This position provides a primary window to logical and emotional understanding and memory, motor planning of the lower extremities, and sensorimotor integration. Secondary functions include word recognition, auditory processing, recognition of faces and symbols, running, walking kicking, and ambulation.

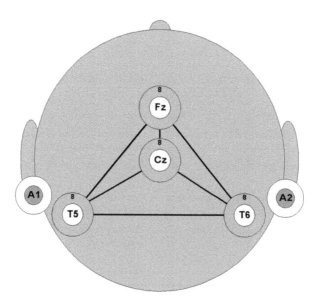

Figure 12.11 Sites: T5 T6 Fz Cz "Posterior Temporal and Frontal Midline."

10-20 territory modules	Principal function	Other functions
T5	Logical (verbal) understanding	Word recognition Auditory processing
T6	Emotional understanding	Facial recognition Symbol recognition Auditory processing
Fz	Motor planning of both lower extremities (BLE) and midline	Running, walking, kicking
Cz	Sensorimotor integration both lower extremities (BLE) and midline	Ambulation

Coherence	Result of hypo-coherence	Result of hyper-coherence
T5-T6	Less efficient logical memory/emotional memory	Lack of flexibility of logical memory/emotional memory
T5-Fz	Less efficient logical memory/midline motor actions	Lack of flexibility of logical memory/midline motor actions
T5-Cz	Less efficient logical memory/midline sensorimotor integration	Lack of flexibility of logical memory/midline sensorimotor integration
T6-Fz	Less efficient emotional memory/midline motor actions	Lack of flexibility of emotional memory/midline motor actions
T6-Cz	Less efficient emotional memory/midline sensorimotor integration	Lack of flexibility of emotional memory/midline sensorimotor integration
Fz-Cz	Less efficient midline motor action/midline sensorimotor integration	Lack of flexibility of midline motor action/midline sensorimotor integration

Source: Based on Walker et al. (2007)

13

PHOTIC STIMULATION
AND NON-VOLITIONAL
NEUROFEEDBACK

Portions of this chapter are adaptded from Collura and Siever (2009).

If the language of the brain lies in its neuronal coding, then the expression of the brain lies in its rhythmicity and timing. This rhythmicity is due to the selective synchronization and desynchronization of the encoding within billions of pools of neurons that provide the sensory activity of everything that is sensed, thought, or done. Berger (1929) observed all four main rhythms, the alpha, beta, theta, and delta, in his very first EEG recording. It should come as no surprise, therefore, that since the earliest EEG studies, interest has turned toward rhythmic sensory stimulation and its possible effects on brain function.

Auditory or visual stimulation can take a wide variety of forms, generating different subjective and clinical effects. The simplest form of stimulation is to present a series of light flashes or sound clicks at a particular rate to a subject and investigate the resulting subjective or EEG effects. This "open-loop" stimulation is not contingent on the EEG brain-wave in any way. From this basic form, changes can be made in the type of stimulation without dependence on the EEG waves.

Clinical reports of flicker stimulation appear as far back as the dawn of modern medicine. The earliest report of the clinical effect of photic stimulation (c. 1900) was described by Pieron (1982), who described the experience of clinicians at the Saltpietre Hospital in Paris. They were exposed to a kerosene lantern whose light was interrupted by a rotating, spoked wheel by a Dr. Pierre Janet. They experienced a reduction in depression, tension, and hysteria. With the development of the EEG, Adrian and Matthews published their results showing that the alpha rhythm could be "driven" above and below the natural frequency with photic stimulation (Adrian and Matthews, 1934). This discovery prompted several small physiological outcome studies on the "flicker following response," the brain's electrical response to stimulation (Bartley, 1934, 1937; Durup and Fessard, 1935; Jasper, 1936; Goldman et al., 1938; Jung, 1939; Toman, 1941).

In the "open-loop" system of visual stimulation, flickering or flashing light can be replaced with sinewave and other types of modulated light. Generally, the more elaborate the photic stimulation, the greater the potential for the brain to interpret and respond. For example, sinewave-modulated light has a significantly greater effect on endogenous rhythms than a simple flickering light. In the case of auditory stimulation, simple clicks can be replaced with modulated or "warbling" sounds, or with binaurally presented "beats." In the case of binaural beats, two different signals are presented to each ear, and the reconstruction of the frequency difference or "beat" is performed within the brain itself.

It is also possible to introduce dependence of the stimulation on the EEG wave so that it becomes EEG-driven, or "closed-loop," or "contingent." Contingent stimulation is produced when the parameters of the feedback are determined by the properties of the EEG. There are a variety of ways to achieve closed-loop control of feedback. These include both direct (phase-sensitive) and indirect (frequency- or amplitude-sensitive) methods. Contingent stimulation greatly increases the possibility for learning to occur, and learning may even occur without conscious effort ("volition"). When the brain is presented with information, including stimulation, that reflects EEG information, the possibilities for classical conditioning, operant conditioning, concurrent learning, and self-efficacy arise. There are a variety of ways to make the stimulation contingent on the EEG, and these include approaches described by Carter et al. (1999), Davis (2005) and Collura (2005). These methods can be broken into two types: phase-sensitive and frequency-sensitive. In phase-sensitive feedback, the photic stimulation is determined by the exact details of the EEG wave, including the timing of peaks and valleys (Davis, 2005).

As EEG equipment improved, so did a renewed interest in the brain's evoked electrical response to photic and auditory stimulation, and soon a flurry of studies were completed (Chatrian et al., 1959; Barlow, 1960; Van der Tweel and Lunel, 1965; Kinney et al., 1973; Townsend, 1973; Donker et al., 1978; Frederick et al., 1999).

Published work in AVS tends to fall into one of three categories: (1) subjective experiential effects of AVS; (2) EEG changes associated with AVS with possible diagnostic value; and (3) clinical applications of AVS. The first type of work has been reported by Huxley (1963), Budzynski and Tang (1998), and others. These have shown that rhythmic information can produce unique sensory experiences associated with the properties of the stimulation. These can include sensations, such as activation, relaxation, or discomfort, visual experiences, and "twilight" states.

Aldous Huxley (1963) was among the first to articulate the subjective correlates of what he described as the "stroboscopic lamp." In his view, "we descend from chemistry to the still more elementary realm of physics. Its rhythmically flashing light seems to act directly, through the optic nerves, on the electrical manifestations of the brain's activity." He described subjective experiences of incessantly changing patterns whose color was a function of the rate of flashing. Between 10 and 15 flashes per second, he reported orange and red; above 15, green and blue; above 18, white and grey. He also described enriched and intensified experiences when subjects were under the effects of mescaline or lysergic acid. In his view, the rhythms of the lamp interacted with the rhythms of the brain's electrical activity to produce a complex interference pattern that is translated by the brain's apparatus into a conscious pattern of color and movement. He remained mystified, however, by one subject who reported seeing an abstract geometry described as a "Japanese landscape" of surpassing beauty, charged with preternatural light and color. Clearly, this simple procedure elicited brain responses far more complex than a simple interference pattern involving basic rhythmic interactions. It comprises the first report of the subjective responses to a simple, non-contingent stimulation.

The second type of work is reported by Walter and Walter (1949), Regan (1989), Collura (2001a), Silberstein (1995), and Frederick et al. (2004). These studies have shown that the EEG can produce both transient and lasting changes as a result of the stimulation. Collura (1978a) articulated the relationship between the low-frequency and high-frequency components of the steady-state visual evoked potential as reflecting anatomically and physiologically distinct response mechanisms, and also demonstrated that the short-term waxing and waning in the steady-state visual evoked response reflects short-term changes in attention.

Srinivarsan (1988) described a direct method in which the intensity of the photic stimulation was directly related to the instantaneous amplitude of the subject's EEG alpha wave. The stimulation was thus both phase locked to, and proportional to the size of, the alpha signal. He reported enhanced alpha amplitude when subjects attended to the stimulator, with concomitant subjective reports consistent with enhanced alpha activity. Systems such as these do not appeal to any need for operant conditioning or for instructions to the test subject. These methods are thus deemed "non-volitional," in that they do not depend on the volition (intent) of the subject. Collura (2005) has further described a non-volitional method that employs selective photic stimulation at a predetermined flicker frequency, but which is presented contingent on the EEG meeting certain criteria. This approach can be used to inhibit particular EEG rhythms, and is also a non-volitional method.

The following single-session example demonstrates the capability of EEG-controlled photic stimulation when applied in an extinction-learning model to reduce excess theta activity. The trainee complained of not being able to control the level of his or her theta, and that it was known to be in excess in previous EEG analyses. The sensor was placed at Oz, and a single channel of EEG was used. The method was based on Collura (2005) as a means of reducing the theta activity by non-volitional EEG-controlled training. The following results were obtained using a five-minute photic training period beginning at minute 30, with no additional instructions given to the trainee.

Figure 13.1 shows the amplitude of theta (4.0–7.0 Hz) as a function of time during a test session. Minutes 1–30: conventional neurofeedback. Minute 30: contingent photic stimulation (14 Hz peripheral white LEDs flashed when theta > threshold) begins. Minute 35: contingent photic stimulation is withdrawn. The continued effect of the learned extinction is evident. Minute 47: trainee is talking. Motion artifact is present.

The initial 30 minutes of monitoring showed the expected high levels of theta, averaging above 20 microvolts peak-to-peak. During this time, conventional feedback was presented in the form of bar graphs and sounds indicating when theta was below a threshold. At minute 31, photic stimulation was introduced so that flashes at 14 per second were delivered whenever the momentary theta value exceeded a second threshold value. For the next five minutes, the trainee experienced the intermittent 14 Hz photic stimulation in both eyes, using peripheral LED glasses so that the trainee could continue to watch the EEG biofeedback display. At minute 35, the stimulation was discontinued and the trainee continued to watch the neurofeedback display, as before.

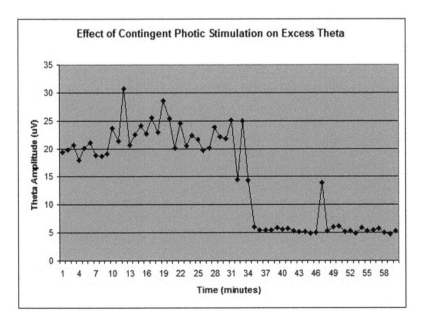

Figure 13.1 Results from a single session using contingent photic stimulation targeting excess theta.

Figure 13.1 shows that the theta amplitude changed abruptly, from its standing level of over 20 microvolts to a level below 10 microvolts within the five-minute learning period. Moreover, the theta amplitude remains at the new level well after the removal of the stimulation and does not show any tendency to recover, or "creep up," for the remainder of the session. The "blip" at minute 47 occurs when the trainee is talking, basically remarking that "my theta level is staying down."

It appears from these results that the effect of the five-minute learning interval was to produce a sustained change in theta activity that persisted well after the stimulation was withdrawn. Therefore, in contrast to "open-loop" stimulation, this method produces a robust and clear learning effect that is lasting. Furthermore, this learning did not depend on intention, as the trainee was given no instructions. Rather, the training was non-volitional. The learning process was thus a result of intrinsic brain processes mediating the change directly as a result of the effect of the stimulation on theta production.

Although photic stimulation can be shown to produce subjective effects as a result of cortical stimulation, it is another issue entirely to conclude that it interacts with, or produces, endogenous rhythms. If, for example, a light flashing at 10 flashes per second produces EEG responses at 10 cycles per second, this does not imply that the flashing is producing an "alpha" rhythm. Endogenous rhythms are associated with particular thalamo-cortical and cortico-cortical mechanisms, and are self-sustaining (Sterman, 1996). Responses to flickering light, on the other hand, are produced by the same mechanisms that produce simple evoked potentials, and thus involve sensory and perceptual mechanisms that are different from the innate cortical rhythmic generators. This is confirmed by the fact that photic "entrainment" effects in the EEG are invariably seen to vanish when the stimulation is withdrawn. In other words, the EEG is not "entrained" in the sense of "driving" an alpha rhythm. Rather, a repetitive evoked potential is produced whose frequency content is simply related to the frequency of the stimulating flashes. However, the presence of these frequencies reflects an entirely different mechanism and functional anatomical basis when compared with endogenous rhythms.

Harmonics are also commonly seen in the EEG responses to photic stimulation. Again, these do not need to be interpreted as "beta" or "gamma" rhythms produced by the stimulation. Rather, the presence of higher harmonics is understood as a simple product of the complex waveform that is elicited. True beta, gamma, and similar high-frequency EEG rhythms are produced by particular cortico-cortical mechanisms and are modulated as a function of cortical excitability. When a visual evoked response is produced, it has its own low-frequency and high-frequency components, regardless of the frequency of stimulation. The high-frequency components are the primary cortical responses, and low-frequency components reflect secondary cortical mechanisms. It so happens that when the stimulation occurs at certain rates, the overlapping of the separate evoked potential components reinforces a particular component due to the linear superposition of the waveforms. Thus, the frequencies elicited by repetitive stimulation reflect different neuronal mechanisms than those producing the endogenous rhythms.

As a result, the benefits of AVS are not simple or "automatic." That is, by stimulating at or near the alpha frequency, for example, we should not expect to elicit the same effects as the brain producing its endogenous alpha rhythm. There may be subjective correlates to the stimulation that resemble an alpha state, but this is not an intrinsic alpha state. In furthering the field, both the short-term and long-term EEG and clinical effects of the stimulation must be studied in order to produce a coherent scientific and clinical rationale.

This chapter explores and analyzes methods for using repetitive or rhythmic stimulation in the context of EEG neurofeedback protocols. Basic principles and examples using event-related potentials as biofeedback signals have been described by Rosenfeld et al. (1984). A key issue is the real-time extraction and feedback of relevant evoked potential information. There are many ways to introduce such stimulation into a neurofeed-back setting, and different approaches have different effects on the training, the subject, and the outcome. We will show results of pilot studies using flickering (pulsed) light stimulation to produce an EEG response. The focus is on instrumentation, methods, and underlying physiological concepts. While the literature contains a variety of clinical reports on therapeutic effects (for example, Patrick, 1996), the purpose here is to identify key methodologies and review their applicability from a basic point of view.

Whenever a brief stimulus is presented to a trainee, there is a transient brain response due to that stimulation (Ciganek, 1961). The signal produced in the EEG is generally very small, but it can be detected. In cases where it is possible to discern the EEG changes, either in the raw EEG or in a processed form, then there is said to be an *event-related potential* (ERP), particularly a *sensory evoked potential*. The evoked potential provides an indication of the effect of the stimulus on the brain, and it has been established that the EP is sensitive to changes in sensory and perceptual processes (Schechter and Buchsbaum, 1973; Naatanen, 1975).

Stimulation may be repetitive or it may be non-repetitive. By repetitive, we mean that successive stimuli occur within a relatively short interval of time (well below one second), they occur at regular intervals, and they are sustained throughout the stimulation period, which can be anywhere from under a second, to many minutes, or more. When the stimulation is not repetitive, then it is said that there is a single EEG brain evoked potential response that is embedded in the ongoing EEG activity. If the stimuli are provided in a successive manner so that a computer can analyze more than one of them, it is possible to extract an estimate of the averaged evoked potential, which represents a canonical, or standard, response of the brain to the stimuli. When the stimulation is repetitive in nature, each stimulus follows the previous one by a short period of time (less than 500 milliseconds), and the successive evoked responses in the brain are found to overlap in time so that the trailing end of one response is superimposed upon the beginning of the next.

When repetitive stimulation is applied, there is a small periodic signal introduced in the EEG. This phenomenon was first reported by Walter and Walter (1949). Studies by Van der Tweel and Lunel (1965) and Regan (1966) further clarified this effect. In general, a repetitive flash produces an EEG response at the same frequency as the stimulation, and harmonics may be present. When sinusoidal light is applied, there is a stabilizing effect and an interaction with intrinsic rhythms (Townsend et al., 1975). This is not seen in the case of flickering or square-wave light, which produces a simple train of stimulus-induced visual evoked potential waves (Sato et al., 1971; Kinney et al., 1973). Van Hof (1960) analyzed averaged visual evoked responses to a flash stimulus and compared the waveform produced by repetitive flashes to that predicted by arithmetically combining the response to flashes at 1 per second. The linearity of overlap was confirmed by showing this equivalence for the entire range of flash rate studied, with flash rates of 2 per second to 18 per second. Childers and Perry (1971) presented averaged visual evoked response elicited by spot flashes from 0.5 per second to 15 per second. Visual inspection of their waveforms confirms that the size and latency of evoked potential components is preserved across frequencies, and that the successive responses overlap, producing the observed response. Furthermore, the synchronous component response shown in their report is identical in shape to the frequency spectrum of single evoked responses presented by McGillem and Aunon (1977). This similarity in spectral energy distribution is what would be expected from a linear overlap model (Collura, 1987, 1990). In particular, a low-frequency band of 4–10 Hz is evident, and a higher-frequency band of 12–20 Hz is also evident. From these results, it is clear that repetitive visual stimulation produces a periodic evoked potential in the EEG, and that the frequency characteristics of this periodic wave can be predicted by using simple linear superposition.

Flickering and square-wave light are understood to produce results by similar mechanisms, although square-wave stimulation produces separate "on" and "off" responses, which are combined in the case of a single momentary "on/off" response to a brief light flash. Despite this difference, observations with both flicker and square-wave evoked potentials can be entirely explained by the assumption that evoked responses are being elicited in a repetitive manner based upon linear superposition of the responses. This includes the presence of harmonics, which are a simple consequence of the complex wave shape of the individual evoked responses and the resulting Fourier series that describes the frequency spectrum (Collura, 1978a, 1990). This point of view is further supported by work reported by Saltzberg (1976), which shows that transient wavelets in the EEG produce measurable peaks in EEG spectral power that can be observed in the frequency spectrum. Based upon this understanding, our laboratory works exclusively with flicker and square-wave stimuli, and analyzes the EEG in narrow frequency bands. It follows from the mathematics of linear superposition that slow EP components will be manifested in the lowest (fundamental) response, while faster components will be reflected in higher (second and higher harmonic) frequencies.

Further rationale for using this approach in neurofeedback includes the observation that transient evoked potentials exhibit correlations with attention and mental task (Spong et al., 1969). Evoked potentials also show systematic differences in clinical populations, particularly with regard to ADD and ADHD. Linden et al. (1996) showed that an ADHD group had abnormal high amplitude early components of the VEP, and that a mixed group (ADD and ADD/ADHD) had slow latency late components (N2, P3). Lubar (1991) reported similar findings in the 300–500-millisecond post-stimulus responses for LD children compared to normals. Further results were reported by Barabasz et al. (1999), who saw delayed P300s in children with ADD and ADHD. These findings are consistent with the high theta/low beta/SMR profile of such children, based on the under-standing that the speed of cortical response is one factor that determines the frequency distribution of an EEG rhythm. This suggests that SSVEP latencies and amplitudes can be important indicators for assessment, as well as for training. In the interest of pursuing real-time feedback of SSVEP information, we recorded EEG and SSVEP traces under different attentive tasks to demonstrate systematic differences.

The relationship between late ERP components and endogenous rhythms becomes clear if one considers the commonalities, as well as the differences, between evoked and intrinsically generated cortical activity. In the case of endogenous rhythms, interaction between the cortical centers and the thalamic nuclei produce interactive sequences of afferent and efferent bursts, which are accompanied by sequences of cortical responses. In essence, an endogenous rhythm consists of a train of "intrinsic evoked potentials," which are elicited by thalamo-cortical interaction, rather than by sensory stimulation. A sensory evoked potential, on the other hand, consists of the cortical response to a particular sensory input that is specified in time. In both cases, the frequency characteristics of the individual cortical responses become manifested in the power spectral density of the resulting EEG wave (Collura, 1987). Since later components of individual cortical responses produce lower frequencies in the composite power spectrum, it is reasonable to expect a cortex that produces increased or delayed late components in a sensory evoked potential to also show increased energy in low frequencies in endogenous EEG activity.

To further understand the origin of the SSVEP waves, refer to Figures 13.2 and 13.3. These show the anatomic pathways involved in the processing of visual information (Brodal, 1969; Regan, 1989). Note, in particular, that afferent neural signals originating in the retina of the eye are first sent to thalamic nuclei, where they are preprocessed, and then forwarded to the occipital and infero-temporal cortexes, before being sent to other cortical locations. The initial processing in Brodman's areas 17 and 18 leads to the early components of the evoked response (less than 150 milliseconds), and further processing in other cortical locations produces the later components (200 to 400 milliseconds). This was illustrated, for example, in trauma studies by Greenberg et al. (1977), in which loss of primary visual areas resulted in decreased or extinguished fast EP components, while loss of secondary areas resulted in decreased or extinguished slower components. In terms of the SSVEP, it can be shown that the early components will lead to higher frequency terms in the SSVEP (above 12 Hz) and the later components will lead to lower frequency terms (10 Hz and below) (McGillem and Aunon, 1977; Collura, 1987). These

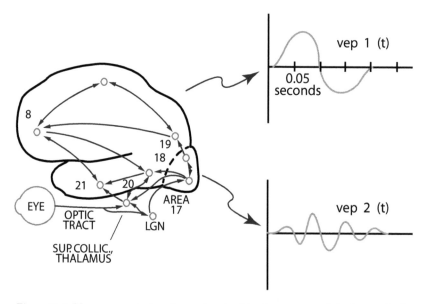

Figure 13.2 Neuroanatomical pathways involved in the response of the human brain to a light flash. When the neural activity first reaches the visual cortex, Brodman areas 17 and 18, the early components of the visual evoked potential are produced. As activity diffuses in the cortex and reaches the association areas, the later components of the evoked potential are produced.

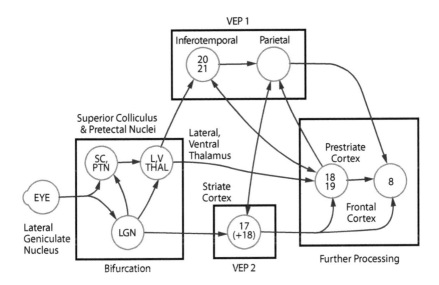

Figure 13.3 Anatomical pathways involved in the response to a visual stimulus.

components are thus visible in the filter outputs of a system that stimulates at a predetermined repetitive rate (e.g. 7 Hz) and filters at both the fundamental and the harmonic of that rate (e.g. 14 Hz).

In addition to clarifying the anatomical sources of the EP waves, this analysis helps to distinguish "driven" rhythms from endogenous rhythms, which are described by Sterman (1996) and Lubar (1997). Whereas the former are mediated by sensory/perceptual mechanisms and are synchronized to the incoming stimulation, endogenous rhythms are self-paced and involve a complex interaction between the cortex and the thalamus. As a result, short-term variations in amplitude and frequency of endogenous rhythms are mediated by different mechanisms than sensory evoked potentials. One potential commonality that exists between the two is the involvement of the cortical response, which partially determines the amplitude and shape of the rhythmic EEG activity, whether it is responding to repetitive sensory stimulation or to intrinsically controlled pacemaker activity.

Figure 13.4 shows the signal relationships between the transient EP, the repetitive stimulation, the steady-state response, and the frequency spectra of each. The top traces represent a single EP and its corresponding frequency spectrum. This is portrayed in the form shown by Childers and Perry (1971) and McGillem and Aunon (1977). The middle traces portray the repetitive stimulus as a train of impulse functions and their frequency spectrum. This spectrum is a train of impulses in the frequency domain (Brigham, 1974). The bottom traces show the repetitive evoked potential and its frequency

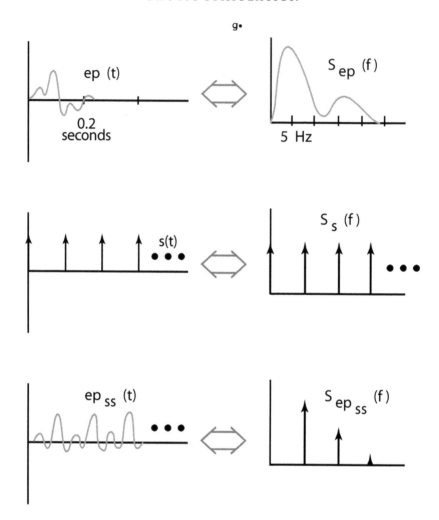

Figure 13.4 Signal and frequency spectral properties of a visual evoked potential (VEP), a repetitive stimulus train, and the resulting steady-state visual evoked potential (SSVEP). Left traces: time-domain signals. Right traces: corresponding frequency spectra (magnitude of the Fourier Transform). Top traces: single VEP and its spectrum. Middle traces: stimulus train and its spectrum. Bottom traces: SSVEP and its spectrum. All right-hand traces are Fourier Transforms of the corresponding left-hand traces. The bottom left signal is the convolution of the two signal above it, while the bottom right spectrum is the product of the two spectra above it, due to the convolution theorem of the Fourier Transform. This analysis explains the observed EEG spectral peaks at the fundamental and harmonic frequencies when a repetitive visual stimulus is presented.

spectrum. The evoked response is given by the convolution of the single EP and the input train, and the spectrum of the evoked response is given by the product of the corresponding spectra of the single response and the stimulus train as a result of the convolution theorem of the Fourier Transform (Oppenheim and Schafer, 1975). Because of this frequency-domain multiplication, the spectrum of the SSVEP is essentially a sampled version of the spectrum of the individual EPs, thus providing an estimate of the size of the peaks of the top spectrum, at frequencies defined by the rate of stimulation, and its integral harmonics. This analysis demonstrates that while the rate of stimulation determines the frequencies at which SSVEP energy will exist, the morphology of the individual EP responses determines the amplitude of those peaks, and also introduces the short-term variations in response amplitude.

The SSVEP can be recorded by filtering the EEG using narrow-band filters. The filters are designed with center frequencies that match the stimulus frequency and its integral harmonics. This provides the ability to measure the signal components in real time. By reconstructing the periodic waveform from its harmonic components, the entire SSVEP can be estimated. The underlying signal model and method of measurement has been described by Collura and Lorig (1977) and Collura (1978a, 1990, 1996). This method focuses on analyzing the EEG components that are locked to the stimulus, and is designed to reject other activity. Thus, this method does not attempt to determine any effects that the stimulation has on intrinsic rhythms or background activity. Instead, it focuses on measuring the response to the stimulation only, thus reflecting sensory/perceptual activity both from primary sensory areas and also any broader cortical late activity that may also be stimulus-locked.

In summary, in order to record evoked potentials in this manner, we stimulate at the rate F flashes per second, and then filter the EEG at 1F, 2F, 3F, and so on. All of the recordings shown here were measured using specially constructed analog filters using standard design methods (Millman and Halkias, 1972). The SSVEP can be measured in real time, and it could be fed back, permitting the trainee to hear the visual cortex as it responds to the lights that are being seen. In the studies shown here, there was no feedback to the trainee.

Subjects in this study were four normal males of college age. They were screened to ensure that none had a psychological or neurological disorder, including epilepsy or ADD. Example data were recorded during a single session for the 4 Hz studies, and another session for the 7.5/8.5 Hz studies. Data shown are typical and illustrative, being from single trials of the methods described below.

Visual stimuli were presented using yellow LEDs mounted in welder's goggles positioned over the subject's open eyes. LEDs were positioned to achieve visual overlap ("fusion") of the two spots. LEDs were driven by

10-millisecond current pulses, providing an averaged light output of 0.0023 milliwatts per eye. A Grass silver chloride electrode was placed at Oz, referenced to the right ear, with a left ear ground. EEG was measured using a Grass Model 12 EEG amplifier (type 7P511) with bandwidth set at 0.1 to 30 Hz. This signal was fed into channel 1 of a Hewlett Packard Signal Averager, which was set to average 64 successive responses. The signal was also sent to a custom-built comb filter that filtered the EEG at 4, 8, 12, and 16 Hz, using third-order analog filters (Butterworth type). The time constant of the filters was set at 2.5 seconds. This provided an effective bandwidth of 0.13 Hz, which is sufficient to reject unrelated EEG activity while responding quickly to changes in the evoked responses. The output of this filter was fed into channel 2 of the signal averager for display, where it could be superimposed on the averaged signal computed within the instrument. Channel 2 was not averaged, however. As channel 1 was collected and averaged, channel 2 was set to free run, providing a single sweep display that synchronized the two signals for visual comparison. Screen images were captured using a Polaroid camera attached to the bezel of the averager.

As an alternative presentation, time series were recorded on a Gould Model 2400 four-channel strip chart recorder. All four banks of the comb filter were summed into one channel of the strip chart to reveal the composite SSVEP as an ongoing waveform. This was plotted simultaneously with the raw EEG signal for visual comparison.

When monitoring short-term state changes, visual stimulation of 8.5 flashes per second was used. Auditory stimulation (clicks) at 7.5 per second was also presented as an alternative target for the subject's attentive focus. EEG was fed into the comb filters described above, with center frequencies set at 7.5, 15, 8.5, and 17 Hz. The output of the comb filters was fed into a Gould Model 2400 four-channel strip chart recorder that used pen and ink to record the traces on moving paper. These traces provide a continuous readout of the filter signals. The chart speed was slowed so that one page of data covered two minutes. Because the traces run slowly, the sinusoidal filter outputs draw a solid area that describes the amplitude (envelope) of the signal. For the 7.5/8.5 Hz recordings, individual filter channels were fed to separate traces so that they could be seen independently.

A typical result of the 4 Hz study, including a comparison with the averaged VEP, is shown in Figure 13.5. What is seen is the response of the brain to a light flashing four times per second. There are two traces superimposed on each of the four graphs. One trace, the smoother of the two, is the "free-running" output of the bank of filters set at 4, 8, 12, and 16 cycles per second. Superimposed on each of these filter responses is the average evoked potential computed by the signal averager.

The responses in Figure 13.5 exhibit the familiar ERP components, including the usual positive and negative transitions. The filter outputs

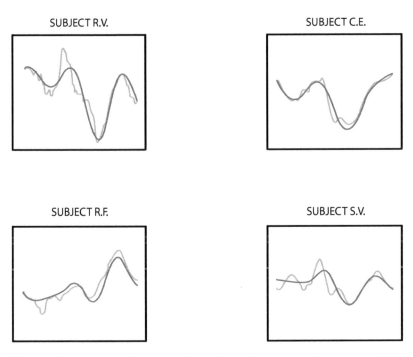

SUBJECT R.V.

SUBJECT C.E.

SUBJECT R.F.

SUBJECT S.V.

Figure 13.5 Superimposed traces for four trials. Each trace contains both the SSVEP (real-time) waveform and the averaged VEP as computed on a computer.

are seen to superimpose on the average evoked potential, demonstrating that, even as we begin to flash repetitively, the resulting wave is a composite evoked potential. During the time that the average is being computed, the filter output was seen to change in shape, as is also evident in Figure 13.4. For example, the bottom right trace of Figure 13.3 (Subject S.V.) shows two leading peaks at approximately 40 and 80 milliseconds in the average, but only one (at approximately 90 milliseconds) in the SSVEP. However, during this acquisition, both peaks were observed in the SSVEP to wax and wane, and also to change in latency; in the final SSVEP sweep, which is the one shown on the display, only the 80 millisecond peak happened to be evident. This illustrates that the SSVEP is capable of dynamically tracking latency (and amplitude) changes that are obscured in the averaged EP, because the averaged EP combines changing features into a single waveform that represents the entire acquisition period. When the average is complete, the screen depicts the final sweep of the filter output, which is an estimate of the most recent SSVEP wave. These time variations are seen more clearly in a continual waveform display, as follows.

Figure 13.6 depicts a subject with an EEG trace running across the top of each pair and the combined output of the filters beneath it. It has been seen that the output of the filters is, in fact, a good estimate of the evoked potential that would be measured with an averager. The benefit of this technique is that the SSVEP is measured in real time, based upon the properties of the filters. Along the top we have the first 16 seconds of the recording. Before the stimulus is presented, the filters have a small output, as seen on the beginning trace. The stimulation is turned on three seconds into this trace. By the time 16 seconds are over, the filters are already producing a very good estimate of the evoked potential. This SSVEP signal consists of a continual series of SSVEP waves that are the same as one trace of Figure 13.3, only shown concatenated in time. The start of each SSVEP wavelet is synchronized with the light flash that is occurring four times per second. If this trace is magnified, it produces an estimate of the waveform that would be obtained from signal averaging. However, instead of waiting a minute or more to see an estimated averaged VEP, it is possible to see the SSVEP result in real time. This output reveals the connection between the transient evoked potential wave morphology and the complex SSVEP wave that consists of the fundamental plus harmonics of the stimulus rate.

On the bottom trace that extends from 32 seconds to 48 seconds after stimulus onset, even though the stimulation period has not approached one

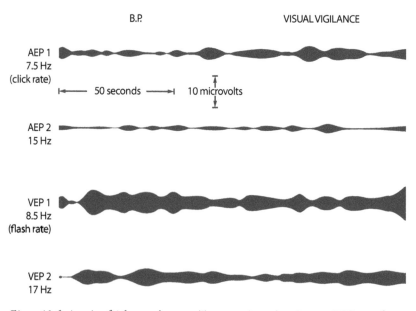

Figure 13.6 A pair of 16-second traces. Top trace in each pair: raw EEG waveform. Bottom trace in each pair: synchronously filtered EEG revealing the time-locked steady-state evoked potential wave. Note time variations in the evoked wave, over periods as small as several seconds.

minute, visible changes are evident. Careful inspection reveals a fine detail in the evoked potentials, and one can identify particular peaks and valleys with particular latencies and amplitudes. These features can be seen changing about every four or five seconds. This method thus allows us to probe the brain functionally, allowing us to see what is occurring live and in real time. This is much different from signal averaging, which provides a single, static wave estimate after a minute or two. The real-time ability of this technique opens the door to doing biofeedback on this type of a response. This is, therefore, EEG evoked potential neurofeedback, and can be performed in real time.

A moment later, the subject performs the corresponding auditory vigilance task (Figure 13.7). There is a visible difference in the time course of the evoked potentials. The entire time here is about two minutes. One can actually see the changes in how the brain responds moment to moment. In the case of auditory vigilance, the visual cortex appears to be much more labile, with much more waxing and waning. The experimental design and statistical results are described in more detail by Collura (1996). These observations are consistent with a sensory gating model, such as that described by Hillyard and Mangoun (1987). Based upon our earlier considerations, these results suggest that the observed variations occur in the attentional pathways that produce the later (lower-frequency) components, rather than in the sensory/perceptual pathways that produce the earlier (higher-frequency) components. This thus provides a very selective mechanism by which we can selectively feed back (and train) the neural pathways of interest, exploiting the signal characteristics as a way to pinpoint the neuroanatomical mechanisms we wish to affect.

We have seen that the response to flashing stimuli produces energy at the fundamental and harmonics of the stimulus rate, and that this is a simple outcome of the generation of a complex periodic wave, which is the SSVEP. It is thus possible to interpret real-time filtered SSVEP data in light of the corresponding EP model. Consider the case with 8.5 stimulation. The response to the 8.5 Hz flash represents the energy in the low-frequency band of McGillem and Aunon (1977), and the 17 Hz response represents the energy in the high-frequency band. We are, in effect, sampling the amplitude of the EP frequency spectrum by performing repetitive stimulation and filtering the corresponding components from the raw EEG. We observe these responses to wax and wane independently, suggesting independent generators in the brain. Our interpretation is that the high-frequency response reflects primary sensory mechanisms that produce short-latency EP components (less than 120 milliseconds) while the low-frequency response reflects secondary mechanisms that produce longer latency (between 150 and 250 milliseconds) components. We are thus able to separate, in frequency, the brain processes that conventional EP averaging endeavors to perform in the time domain. Despite the ease with

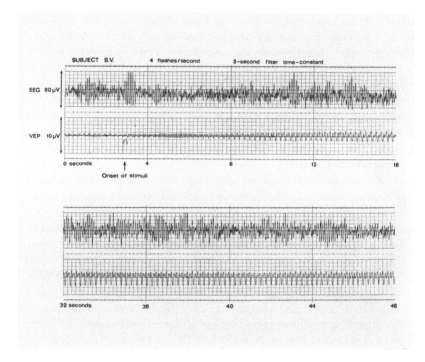

Figure 13.7 SSVEP evoked potential envelopes recorded during a visual vigilance task. Top two traces are auditory responses, and bottom two traces are visual responses. Waxing and waning of the VEP1 component should be noted. In this example, the trainee is performing a visual vigilance task, and is pressing a button whenever a small (less than 3 dB) change is seen in the visual stimulus. The two upper traces show the filtered activity associated with auditory stimulus (clicks), used as an alternative attentive target for the vigilance task. Observing the lower two traces, we see the visual evoked potential at the primary frequency, which happens to be 8.5 Hz. Beneath this is the secondary component at 17 Hz. Visually, a candlestick type of appearance is evident, reflecting the characteristic waxing and waning.

which visually evoked potentials are measured, we saw no such correlate in the auditory realm. Figures 13.5 and 13.6 do not show visually, nor did statistical studies show, that the auditory steady-state evoked potential is sensitive to attention in this type of study.

It should be emphasized that the appearance of harmonics in this case is not due to any non-linearity in the brain. They appear due to the simple signal properties of creating a repetitive signal, which is not just a simple sinewave. The measured EEG response of the brain is what would be predicted if we took the responses to a slower flash and sped them up. It is important to realize this, because there is a tendency to talk about

B.P.   AUDITORY VIGILANCE

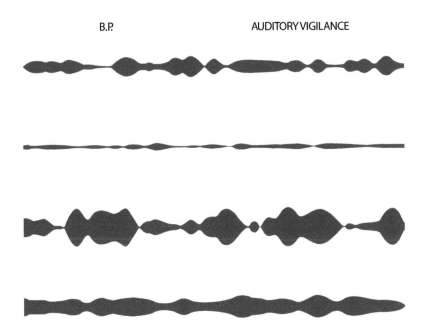

Figure 13.8 SSVEP evoked potential envelopes recorded during an auditory vigilance task. Top two traces are auditory responses, and bottom two traces are visual responses. Waxing and waning of the VEP2 component is noticeably different from Figure 13.5. This illustrates a difference in how the visual attentive mechanisms are responding to the stimulation.

entrainment and driving of brain rhythms, and what we see here is that, electrophysiologically, there is no evidence for any entrainment or EEG driving in this case. Entrainment is a nonlinear, plastic process that would produce: (1) larger than expected evoked responses; and (2) lasting EEG changes after the withdrawal of the stimulus, hopefully for a long period of time. For example, Childers and Perry (1971) argue that their data provide evidence for an alpha "driving" phenomenon, attributed to cortical resonance. However, upon careful inspection, the waveforms presented are as indicative of linear superposition as they are of a resonance phenomenon. Lubar (1998a, 1998b) was motivated to look for both the alpha "resonance" phenomenon and for lasting changes in EEG power spectra at the frequencies of stimulation. In these studies, neither effect was in fact observed.

The entrainment perspective is well articulated by Siever (1997b), which presents EEG traces as evidence for squarewave photic stimuli producing a "frequency following response" that is "most effective" at a rate that matches the natural alpha frequency. The cited traces are, however, entirely consistent with Van Hof (1960), which demonstrated that such traces are, in fact, produced by linear superposition of evoked potential wavelets. Our studies are consistent with Van Hof's, and did not demonstrate any unexpectedly large responses or lasting EEG changes in response to flickering light stimuli. The observed "resonance" at "alpha" is, in fact, an EP response maximum that happens to occupy the same frequencies as low alpha (7–9 Hz). This SSVEP response peak is predictable based upon the morphology of single EPs and the presence of a spectral energy maximum at this range, because the EP itself contains appreciable signal components in the 120- to 140-millisecond range.

There appears to be no direct evidence that repetitive flash stimuli can produce an EEG response that goes beyond the production of a series of transient visually evoked EEG responses. There are various reports and methods that make use of the concept of entrainment in a therapeutic role (Patrick, 1996; Carter et al., 2000). These require model-specific design of equipment and procedures, and appeal to the notion that the frequency of stimulation is tightly coupled of the trainee's endogenous EEG signals and changes therein. Our approach is entirely different. We do not appeal to any notion of entrainment, and our current interests are specifically twofold: to record, measure, and train the sensory pathways that are associated with the evoked activity itself, and to produce EEG systems that are able to control visual stimulation as an assist to neurofeedback, without being restricted to specific frequency or entrainment-based approaches. The evoked potential-based approach appeals to a different set of physiologic considerations, involving the learning processes in sensory-related pathways and interactions between them. These interactions define the nature of the induced SSVEP activity, as well short-term variations in the evoked responses.

How might this be relevant to attention, learning, or task-related performance? One might expect that there would be important differences in the time behavior of these real-time measurements. Previous studies of visual evoked potentials have revealed a systematic dependence on attention and other brain state variables (Naatanen, 1975; Regan, 1989). However, the time course of the relevant mental processes is not revealed by conventional averaged evoked potential techniques.

At the simplest level, photic stimulation can be used with EEG neurofeedback as a simple adjunct. This might precondition an individual before training or postcondition him or her afterwards. This is not integrated with the neurofeedback. This could be used before, during, or after neurofeedback, but it is not controlled by the EEG in any way. However, using the EEG to control the stimulus parameters offers additional possibilities. We are exploring methods that use such control in simple ways. One method is called non-volitional EEG neurofeedback, in which the EEG is used to control a stimulator, generally to train an increase in the evoked response. This approach could also be used to decrease a rhythm.

Simple non-volitional neurofeedback was introduced by Srinivarsan (1988), and Figure 13.9 shows the basic design of this type of system.

Figure 13.10 shows the basic approach to using the SSVEP signal itself for feedback. In a system of this type, the trainee hears the brain's sensory/perceptual response mechanisms in real time, and can use these for training purposes. The audio feedback reflects the brain's response to the repetitive stimulation and allows the trainee to receive feedback regarding his or her current state of attention. This trains different pathways and mechanisms more than conventional neurofeedback. It actually trains the sensory/perceptual pathways based upon evoked activity, using a volitional technique.

It is also possible to perform simple EEG-controlled photostimulation based upon simple control of the light and sound system based on EEG (Figure 13.11). In order to perform EEG-controlled photostimulation, one measures the EEG and filters it, then adds control logic to turn the lights on and off under control of the EEG. This can be used to stimulate at a fixed frequency that has no particular relationship to the endogenous EEG. Initial trials using this method have shown that it may provide a useful assist. The system can turn the stimulators on or off, and can add

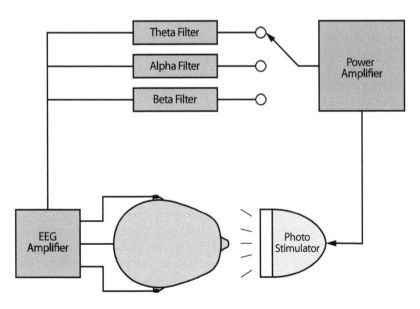

Nonvolitional EEG Biofeedback

Figure 13.9 Basic system for non-volitional EEG biofeedback (after Srinivarsan, 1988). The EEG signal is filtered and used to control a photic stimulator.

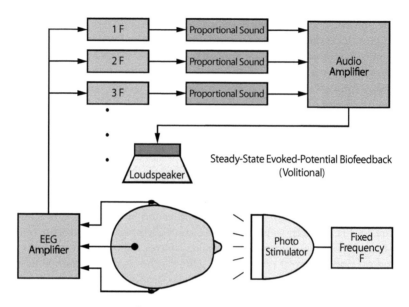

Figure 13.10 Basic system for SSVEP biofeedback. The trainee is photically stimulated at a fixed frequency and the resulting EEG response is measured using comb filters. This information is fed back to the trainee in the form of variable tones.

a non-volitional aspect to enhance the neurofeedback experience. For example, if a 12-flash-per-second stimulation is delivered whenever the subject's theta (4–7 Hz) wave exceeds a threshold value, the system has an effect of extinguishing excessive EEG theta by the simple mechanism of distracting and engaging the cortex so that theta cannot be produced at such a large level.

One can make a distinction between volitional and non-volitional methods using this approach. A volitional method requires instructions to the trainee and presupposes expectation of a reward or a goal. The feedback provides information that must be rapid, accurate, and aesthetic. The trainee must find and recognize states reflected in the feedback information, consciously or unconsciously. Learning occurs with practice under an operant conditioning model and generally produces lasting effects.

In non-volitional methods, on the other hand, there are no instructions to the trainee and the stimulus itself introduces a state or a change in a state. It may introduce the brain to a state, or it may remove the brain from a state. One example of this is theta blocking, described previously. In this case, the effect of the stimulation does not depend on instructions to, or the intent of, the trainee. In time, the trainee may become more accustomed to being in a different brain state. This type of learning is closer to classical conditioning than operant conditioning.

242

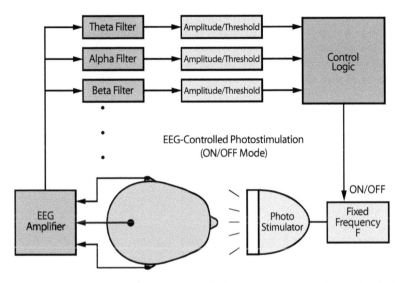

Figure 13.11 Basic system for EEG-controlled photostimulation. Photic stimulation occurs at a set frequency. Based upon a control protocol, the EEG system activates and deactivates the photic stimulation for a variety of uses.

In all of these examples, regardless of volitional or non-volitional aspects of the neurofeedback design, the direct effect of the stimulus on the EEG is transient and disappears once the stimulation is withdrawn. It is thus possible to introduce the brain to a frequency experience, and, after a brief period of this experience, discontinue the stimulation. Such methods may reduce neurofeedback training times, but do not depend on any determination of the dominant EEG frequencies or appeal to any nonlinear entrainment phenomena. When we combine volitional and non-volitional neurofeedback, we may be able to produce a more rapid initial ramp-up to the learning process. We can provide an ongoing assist ("training wheels"), or we can assist with difficult aspects; for example, a trainee having difficulty with theta reduction. This can provide more aggressive reduction of undesirable rhythms, can introduce the brain to particular states, and may combine such effects in a single neurofeedback protocol.

This chapter has outlined some specific issues and technical aspects of using repetitive stimulation in conjunction with EEG neurofeedback methods. Repetitive stimulation introduces a periodic evoked response in the EEG that can be measured and fed back in real time. It is shown that these methods provide an extension of classical EP methods, introducing a real-time aspect. As a result, when we use repetitive stimulation with neurofeedback, there are a range of possible methods and configurations, many of which remain to be explored. We can add non-volitional aspects to the volitional neurofeedback, which may have significant effects. We can also probe specific brain pathways and mechanisms. It is clear that we have just begun to scratch the surface, and considerable research and development should be anticipated before we have explored all of the possibilities that are apparent.

BIBLIOGRAPHY

Adrian, E. and Matthews, B. (1934) "The Berger rhythm: potential changes from the occipital lobes in man," *Brain*, 57: 355–384.

Alshab, A., Collura, T. F., and Voltz, M. D. (2005) "Predicting alertness with EEG processing in patients undergoing deep brain stimulator placement for Parkinson's disease," *Proceedings of the American Society for Anesthesia Annual Meeting*, 651385.

Arns, M., Drinkenburg, W., and Kenemans, J. L. (2012) "The effects of QEEG-informed neurofeedback in ADHD: an open-label pilot study," *Applied Psychophysiology and Biofeedback*, DOI 10.1007/s10484-012-9191-4.

Arns, M., de Ridder, S., Strehl, U., Bretelet, M., and Coenen, A. (2009) "Efficacy of neurofeedback treatment in ADHD: the effects on inattention, impulsivity and hyperactivity: a meta-analysis," *Clinical EEG and Neuroscience*, 40(3): 180–189.

Ayers, M. E. (1999) "Assessing and treating open head trauma, coma, and stroke using real-time digital EEG neurofeedback," in J. R. Evans and A. Abarbanel (Eds.) *Introduction to Quantitative EEG and Neurofeedback*, New York: Academic Press, pp. 203–222.

Baehr, E. and Rosenfeld, J. P. (2001) "Clinical use of an alpha asymmetry neurofeedback protocol in the treatment of mood disorders: follow-up study one to five years post therapy," *Journal of Neurotherapy*, 4(4): 11–17.

Baehr, E., Rosenfeld, J., and Baehr, R. (2001) "Clinical use of an alpha asymmetry neurofeedback protocol in the treatment of mood disorders: follow-up study one to five years post therapy," *Journal of Neurotherapy*, 4(4): 11–18.

Barabasz, A., Stevens, R., and Genthe, T. (1999) "Hypnotizability and EEG ERPs in children with and without ADHD," presented at the 50th Annual Workshop and Scientific Program of the Society for Clinical and Experimental Hypnosis, New Orleans, November 11–14.

Barlow, J. (1960) "Rhythmic activity induced by photic stimulation in relation to intrinsic alpha activity of the brain in man," *Electroencephalography and Clinical Neurophysiology*, 12: 317–326.

Bartley, S. (1934) "Relation of intensity and duration of brief retinal stimulation by light to the electrical response of the optic cortex of the rabbit," *American Journal of Physiology*, 108: 307–408.

Bartley, S. (1937) "Some observations on the organization of the retinal response," *American Journal of Physiology*, 120: 184–189.

Basar, E. (2005) "Memory as the 'whole brain work'—a large-scale model based on 'oscillations in super-synergy'," *International Journal of Psychophysiology*, 58: 199–236.

Berger, H. (1929) "Ueber das Elektroenkephalogramm des Menschen," *Archiv für Psychiatrie und Nervenkrankheiten*, 87: 527–570.

Birbaumer, N. (1997) "Abstract," 5th Annual Winter Conference on Brain Function/ EEG Modifications and Training, Advanced Meeting/Colloquium, Palm Springs, California.

Birbaumer, N. (2002) *Slow Cortical Potential Biofeedback: A New Form of Neurofeedback, with a Long History of Research Support*, DVD available from Futurehealth, retrieved May 27, 2013 from: www.futurehealth.org/simple/biofeedback-and-locked-in-syndrome-in-40.html/.

Birbaumer, N. (2006) "Breaking the slience: brain-computer interfaces (BCI) for cummunication and motor control," *Psychophysiology*, 43: 517–532.

Birbaumer, N., Elbert, T., Canavan, A. G., and Rochstroh, B. (1990) "Slow potential so the cerebral cortex and behavior," *Physiological Review*, 70(1): 1–41.

Bliokh, P., Nikolaenko, A., and Filippov, Y. (1980) *Schumann Resonances in the Earth-Ionosphere Cavity*, London: Peter Perigrinus.

Breakspear, M. and Williams, L. M. (2004) "A novel method for the topographic analysis of neural activity reveals formation and dissolution of 'dynamic cell assemblies'," *Journal of Computational Neuroscience*, 16: 49–68.

Breteler, M., Arns, M., Peters, S., Giepmans, I., and Verhoeven, L. (2010) "Improvements in spelling after QEEG-based neurofeedback in dyslexia: a randomized controlled treatment study," *Applied Psychophysiology and Biofeedback*, 35(1): 5–11.

Brigham, E. O. (1974) *The Fast Fourier Transform*, Englewood Cliffs, NJ: Prentice Hall.

Brodal, A. (1969) *Neurological Anatomy in Relation to Clinical Medicine*, New York: Oxford University Press.

Brownback, T. (2010) *The Brownback, Mason and Associates Neurofeedback System (BMANS)*, Allentown, PA: Brownback, Mason & Associates.

Budzynski, T. (2007) "AVS and difficult-to-treat disorders," Proceedings of the 2nd Symposium on Music, Rhythm, and the Brain, Stanford University, Stanford, CA.

Budzynski, T. and Tang, J. (1998) "Biolight effects on the EEG," *SynchroMed Report*, Seattle, WA.

Budzynski, T. and Budzynski, H. (2001) "Brain brightening—preliminary report, December 2001," in-house manuscript, Mind Alive, Edmonton, Alberta, Canada.

Budzynski, T. H., Budzynski, H. K., Evans, J. R., and Abarbanal, A. (2005) *Introduction to Quantitative EEG and Neurofeedback*, Amsterdam: Elsevier.

Budzynski, T., Jordy, J., Budzynski, H. K., Tang, H. Y., and Claypoole, K. (1989) "Academic performance enhancement with photic stimulation and EDR feedback," *Journal of Neurotherapy*, 3(3).

Burgess, R. and Collura, T. F. (1992) "Polarity, localization, and field determination in electroencephalography," in E. Wyllie (Ed.) *The Treatment of Epilepsy: Principles and Practice*, Philadelphia, PA: Lea & Feiberger, pp. 211–233.

Calvin, W. H. (1989) *The Cerebral Symphony*, New York: Bantam Books.

Cannon, R. and Lubar, J. (2007) "EEG spectral power and coherence: differentiating effects of spatial-specific neuro-operant learning (SSNOL) utilizing LORETA neurofeedback training in the anterior cingulate and bilateral dorsolateral prefrontal cortices," *Journal of Neurotherapy*, 11(3): 25–44.

Cannon, R., Lubar, J., Sokhadze, E., and Baldwin, D. (2008) "LORETA neurofeedback for addiction and the possible neurophysiology of psychological processes influenced:

a case study and region of interest analysis of LORETA neurofeedback in right anterior cingulate cortex," *Journal of Neurotherapy*, 12(4): 227–241.

Cannon, R., Congedo, M., Lubar, J., and Hutchens, T. (2009) "Differentiating a network of executive attention: LORETA neurofeedback in anterior cingulate and dorsolateral prefrontal cortices," *International Journal of Neuroscience*, 119(3): 404–441.

Cannon, R., Lubar, J., Thornton, K., Wilson, S., and Congedo, M. (2005) "Limbic beta activation and LORETA: can hippocampal and related limbic activity be recorded and changes visualized using LORETA in an affective memory condition?" *Journal of Neurotherapy*, 8(4): 5–24.

Cannon, R., Lubar, J., Gerke, A., Thornton, K., Hutchens, T., and McCammon, V. (2006a) "EEG spectral power and coherence: LORETA neurofeedback training in the anterior cingulate gyrus," *Journal of Neurotherapy*, 10(1): 5–31.

Cannon, R., Lubar, J. F., Congedo, M., Gerke, A., Thornton, K., Kelsay, B., et al. (2006b) "The effects of neurofeedback training in the cognitive division of the anterior cingulate gyrus," *International Journal of Science* (in press).

Carter, G. C. (1987) "Coherence and time delay estimation," *Proceedings of the Institute of Electrical and Electronics Engineering*, 75: 236–255.

Carter, J. L. and Russell, H. L. (1993) "A pilot investigation of auditory and visual entrainment of brain wave activity in learning disabled boys," *Texas Researcher*, 4: 65–72.

Carter, J. L., Russell, H. L., and Ochs, L. (1999) "Method and apparatus for changing brain wave frequency," US Patent Number RE36348.

Carter, J. L., Russell, H. L., Vaughn, W. D., and Austin, R. R. (2000) "Method and apparatus for treating an individual using electroencephalographic and cerebral blood flow feedback," US Patent Number 6081743.

Casti, J. L. (1994) *"Complexification": Explaining a Paradoxical World Through the Science of Surprise*, New York: HarperCollins.

Chartier, D., Collins, L., and Koons, D. (1997) "Peak performance EEG training and the game of golf," presented at the 5th Annual Conference on Brain Function/EEG, Palm Springs, CA.

Chatrian, G., Petersen, M., and Lazarte, J. (1959) "Response to clicks from the human brain: some depth electrographic observations," *Electroencephalography and Clinical Neurophysiology*, 12: 479–489.

Childers, D. G. and Perry, N. W. (1971) "Alpha-like activity in vision," *Brain Research*, 25: 1–20.

Ciganek, L. (1961) "The EEG response (evoked potential) to light stimulus in man," *Electroencephalography and Clinical Neurophysiology*, 13: 165–172.

Coben, R. and Evans, J. R. (2011) *Neurofeedback and Neuromodulation Techniques and Applications*, Amsterdam: Elsevier.

Cochran, S. D. (2012) "Corporate peak performance project," *Biofeedback*, 39(3): 123–126.

Cohen, R., Gross, M., and Lazarte, J. (1992) "Preliminary data on the metabolic brain pattern of patients with winter seasonal affective disorder," *Archives of General Psychiatry*, 49: 545–552.

Collura T. F. (1978a) "Synchronous brain evoked potential correlates of directed attention," PhD dissertation, Department of Biomedical Engineering, Case Western Reserve University, Cleveland, OH.

Collura, T. F. (1978b) "Real-time evoked potential correlates of directed attention," *Proceedings of the 31st Annual Conference for Engineering in Medicine and Biology*, Atlanta, GA, October 21–25, p. 10.

Collura, T. F. (1987) "A transient-event model for EEG power spectra," *Proceedings of the 40th Annual Conference for Engineering in Medicine and Biology*, Niagara Falls, NY, September 10–12.

Collura, T. F. (1990) "Real-time filtering for the estimation of steady-state visual evoked brain potentials," *IEEE Transactions on Biomedical Engineering*, 37(6): 650–652.

Collura, T. F. (1996) "Human steady-state visual and auditory evoked potential components during a selective discrimination task," *Journal of Neurotherapy*, 3(1): 1–9.

Collura, T. F. (1999) "Method for self-administration of electroencephalographic (EEG) neurofeedback training," US Patent Number 5899867.

Collura, T. F. (1999) "Steady state evoked potentials—a new channel for EEG biofeedback?" presented at the 1999 Winter Brain Meeting, Palm Springs, CA, February.

Collura, T. F. (2001a) "Application of repetitive visual stimulation to EEG neurofeedback protocols," *Journal of Neurotherapy*, 6(1): 47–70.

Collura, T. F. (2001b) *Coherence Calculation and Quadrature Filtering*, Oakwood Village, OH: BrainMaster Technologies.

Collura, T. F. (2002) "Application of repetitive visual stimulation to EEG neurofeedback protocols," *Journal of Neurotherapy*, 6(2): 47–70.

Collura, T. F. (2005) "System for reduction of undesirable brain wave patterns using selective photic stimulation," US Patent Number 6931275.

Collura, T. F. (2006) "The Atlantis visual/auditory/tactile system," *AVS Journal*, 5(2): 29–32.

Collura, T. F. (2007) "Repetitive visual stimulation to EEG neurofeedback protocols," US Patent Number 7269456.

Collura, T. F. (2009a) "Combining EEG with heart-rate training for brain/body optimization," *NeuroConnections*, Winter: 8–11.

Collura, T. F. (2009b) "Neuronal dynamics in relation to normative electroencephalography assessment and training," *Biofeedback*, 36(4): 134–139.

Collura, T. F. (2009c) "Practicing with multichannel EEG, DC, and slow cortical potentials," *NeuroConnections*, January: 35–39

Collura, T. F. and Lorig, R. J. (1977) "Real-time filtering of transient visual evoked potentials," presented at 30th Annual Conference for Engineering in Medicine and Biology, Los Angeles, CA, November 5–9.

Collura, T. F. and Mrklas, W. (2008) "Multi-channel, multi-variate whole-head normalization using live z-scores," US Patent Application 12/266755; Canadian Patent Number 2643501 pending.

Collura, T. F. and Siever, D. (2009) "Audio-visual entrainment in relation to mental health and EEG," in T. Budzynski, H. K. Budzynski, J. R. Evans, and A. Abarbanal (Eds.) *Quantitative EEG and Neurofeedback* (2nd ed.), San Diego, CA: Academic Press, pp. 155–183.

Collura, T. F., Luders, H., and Burgess, R. C. (1990) "EEG mapping for surgery of epilepsy," *Brain Topography*, 3(1): 65–77.

Collura, T. F., Don, N. S., and Warren, C. A. (2004) "EEG event-related spectral signatures associated with psi-conducive states," presented at the 35th Annual

Meeting of the Association for Applied Psychophysiology and Biofeedback, Colorado Springs, CO, April 1–4.

Collura, T. F., Jacobs, E. C., Braun, D. S., and Burgess, R. C. (1993) "EView—a workstation-based viewer for intensive clinical electroencephalography," *IEEE Transactions on Biomedical Engineering*, 49(9): 736–744.

Collura, T. F., Thatcher, R. W., Smith, M. L., Lambos, W. A., and Stark, C. R. (2009) "EEG biofeedback training using z-scores and a normative database," in W. Evans, T. Budzynski, H. Budzynski, and A. Arbanal (Eds.) *Introduction to QEEG and Neurofeedback: Advanced Theory and Applications* (2nd ed.), New York: Elsevier.

Collura, T. F., Guan, J., Tarrant, J., Bailey, J., and Starr, F. (2010) "EEG biofeedback case studies using live z-score training (LZT) and a normative database," *Journal of Neurotherapy*, 14(2): 22–46.

Congedo, M. (2003) "Tomographic neurofeedback: a new technique for the self regulation of brain electrical activity," unpublished doctoral dissertation, University of Tennessee, Knoxville, TN.

Congedo, M. (2006) "Subspace projection filters for realtime brain electromagnetic imaging," *IEEE Transactions on BioMedical Engineering*, 53: 1624–1634.

Congedo, M., Lubar, J., and Joffe, D. (2004a) "Tomographic neurofeedback: a new technique for the self regulation of brain electrical activity," *Journal of Neurotherapy*, 8(2): 141–142.

Congedo, M., Lubar, J., and Joffe, D. (2004b). "Low resolution electromagnetic tomography neurofeedback," *IEEE Transactions on Neuronal Systems and Rehabilitation Engineering*, 12: 387–397.

Corrigan, N. M., Richards, T., Webb, S. J., Murias, M., Merkle, K., Kleinhans, N. M., et al. (2009) "An investigation into the relationship between fMRI and ERP source localized measurements of brain activity during face processing," *Brain Topography*, 22(2): 83–96.

Davidson, R. J. and Begley, S. (2012) *The Emotional Life of Your Brain*, New York: Penguin Group.

Davis, C. (1999) "The Roshi," personal communication.

Davis, C. (2005) "The pRoshi," personal communication.

Deestexhe, A. and Sejnowski, T. J. (2003) "Interactions between membrane conductances underlying thalamocortical slow-wave oscillations," *Physiological Review*, 83: 1401–1453.

Di Gangi, A. and Birbaumer, N. (2000) "Complexity of brain activity reflects complexity of music," *Proceedings of the European Society for the Cognitive Sciences of Music*, retrieved May 27, 2013 from: www.escom.org/proceedings/ICMPC2000/Tue/Birbaume.htm/.

Donker, D., Njio, L., Storm Van Leewan, W., and Wieneke, G. (1978) "Interhemispheric relationships of responses to sine wave modulated light in normal subjects and patients," *Encephalography and Clinical Neurophysiology*, 44: 479–489.

Durup, G. and Fessard, A. (1935) "L'electroencephalogramme de l'homme" ("The human electroencephalogram"), *Annale Psychologie*, 36: 1–32.

Evans, J. R. (1972) "Multiple simultaneous sensory stimulation of severely retarded children: results of a pilot study," presented at the 1972 meeting of the Southeastern Psychological Association.

Fehmi, L. and Collura, T. (2007) "Effects of electrode placement upon EEG biofeedback training: the monopolar-bipolar controversy," *Journal of Neurotherapy*, 11(2): 45–63.

Fehmi, L. and Robbins, J. (2007) *The Open Focus Brain: Harnessing the Power of Attention to Heal Mind and Body*, Boston, MA: Shambala.

Fehmi, L. L. and Sundor, A. (1989) "The effects of electrode placement upon EEG biofeedback training: the monopolar-bipolar controversy," *International Journal of Psychosomatics*, 36(1–4): 23–33.

Festa, E. K., Heindel, W. C., Connors, N. C., Hirschberg, L., and Ott, B. R. (2009) "Neurofeedback training enhances the efficiency of cortical processing in normal aging," Cognitive Neuroscience Society Annual Meeting Program, A11, p. 41, supplement of the *Journal of Cognitive Neuroscience*.

Fife, D. and Barancik, J. I. (1985) "Northeastern Ohio trauma study, 3: incidence of fractures," *Annual Emergency Medicine*, 14: 244–248.

Fisher, S. (2008) "Neurofeedback and attachment disorder: theory and practice," in T. Budzynski, H. Budzynski, J. E. Evans, and A. Abarbanal (Eds.) *Introduction to Quantitative EEG and Neurofeedback* (2nd ed.), Amsterdam: Elsevier, pp. 315–336.

Fox, P. and Raichle, M. (1985) "Stimulus rate determines regional blood flow in striate cortex," *Annals of Neurology*, 17(3): 303–305.

Frederick, J. A., Timmermann, D. L., Russell, H. L., and Lubar, J. F. (2004) "EEG coherence effects of audio-visual stimulation (AVS) at dominant and twice dominant alpha frequency," *Journal of Neurotherapy*, 8(4): 25–42.

Frederick, J., Lubar, J., Rasey, H., Brim, S., and Blackburn, J. (1999) "Effects of 18.5 Hz audiovisual stimulation on EEG amplitude at the vertex," *Journal of Neurotherapy*, 3(3): 23–27.

Freeman, W. (1991) "The physiology of perception," *Scientific American*, 264(2): 78–85.

Freeman, W. J. (1994a) "Characterization of state transitions in spatially distributed, chaotic, nonlinear, dynamical systems in cerebral cortex," *Integrative Physiological and Behavioral Science*, 29(3): 294–306.

Freeman, W. J. (1994b) "Role of chaotic dynamics in neural plasticity," in J. van Pelt, M. A. Corner, H. B. M. Uylings, and F. H. Lopes da Silva (Eds.) *Progress in Brain Research*, vol. 102, Amsterdam: Elsevier Science, pp. 319–333.

Freeman, W. J., Burke, B. C., and Holmes, M. D. (2003) "Aperiodic phase resetting in scalp EEG of beta-gamma oscillations by state transitions at alpha-theta rates," *Human Brain Mapping*, 19(4): 248–272.

Gagnon, C. and Boersma, F. (1992) "The use of repetitive audio-visual entrainment in the management of chronic pain," *Medical Hypnoanalysis Journal*, 7: 462–468.

Girten, D. G., Benson, K. L., and Kamiya, J. (1973) "Observation of very slow potential oscillations in human scalp recording," *Electroencephalography and Clinical Neurophysiology*, 35: 561–568.

Gleick, J. (1987) *Chaos: Making a New Science*, New York: Penguin Books.

Glicksohn, J. (1986–1987) "Photic driving and altered states of consciousness: an exploratory study," *Imagination, Cognition and Personality*, 6(2): 1986–1987.

Goldman, G., Segal, J., and Segalis, M. (1938) "L'action d'une excitation inermittente sur le rythme de Berger" ("The effects of intermittent excitation on the Berger rhythms (EEG rhythms)"), *C.R. Societe de Biologie Paris*, 127: 1217–1220.

Grave de Peralta Menendez, R. and Gonzalez Andino, S. L. (1999) "Comments on 'Review of methods for solving the EEG inverse problem' by R. D. Pascual-Marqui," *International Journal of Bioelectromagnetism*, 2(1).

Green, R. L. and Ostrander, R. L. (2009) *Neuroanatomy for Students of Behavioral Disorders*, London: W.W. Norton & Co.

Greenberg, R. P., Mayer, D. J., Becker, D. P., and Miller, J. D. (1977) "Evaluation of brain function in severe human head trauma with multimodality evoked potentials," *Journal of Neurosurgery*, 47: 150–177.

Greenblatt, R. E., Ossadtchi, A., and Pflieger, M. E. (2005) "Local linear estimators for the bioelectromagnetic inverse problem," *IEEE Transactions on Signal Processing*, 53(9): 3403–3412.

Gur, R. C., Gur, R. E., Obrist, W., Skolnick, B., and Reivich, M. (1987) "Age and regional blood flow at rest and during cognitive activity," *Archives of General Psychiatry*, 44: 617–621.

Hammond, D. C. (2000) "Neurofeedback treatment of depression with the Roshi," *Journal of Neurotherapy*, 4(2): 45–56.

Hammond, D. C. (2005) "Neurofeedback treatment of depression and anxiety," *Journal of Adult Development*, 12(2/3): 131–137.

Hammond, D. C. and Baehr, E. (2008) "Neurofeedback for the treatment of depression: current status of theoretical issues and clinical research," in T. Budzynski, H. Budzynski, J. E. Evans, and A. Abarbanal (Eds.) *Introduction to Quantitative EEG and Neurofeedback* (2nd ed.), Amsterdam: Elsevier, pp. 241–268.

Hardt, J. V. (1999) Personal communication.

Hardt, J. V. (2001) Personal communication.

Hardt, J. V. and Kamiya, J. (1978) "Anxiety change through electroencephalographic alpha feedback seen only in high anxiety subjects," *Science*, 201: 79–81.

Hartmann, T. (1995) *ADD: A Different Perspective*, Grass Valley, CA: Underwood Books.

Heffernan, M. (1996) "Using chaos to control brainwaves," *Megabrain Report*, 3(1): 14–21.

Henslin, E. (2009) *This is Your Brain on Joy: Revolutionary Programs for Balancing Mood*, Google eBook.

Hillyard, S. A. and Mangoun, G. R. (1987) "Commentary: sensory gating as a physiological mechanism for visual selective attention," in *Current Trends in Event Related Potential Research (EEG Suppl 40)*, Amsterdam: Elsevier Science, pp. 61–67.

Hjorth, B. (1991) "Principles for transformation of scalp EEG from potential field into source distribution," *Journal of Clinical Neurophysiology*, 8(4): 391–396.

Huxley, A. (1963) *The Doors of Perception/Heaven and Hell*, New York: Harper & Row.

Ibric, V. L. and Dragomirescu, L. G. (2008) "Neurofeedback in pain management," in T. Budzynski, H. Budzynski, J. E. Evans, and A. Abarbanal (Eds.) *Introduction to Quantitative EEG and Neurofeedback* (2nd ed.), Amsterdam: Elsevier, pp. 337–364.

Ikeda, A., Luders, H. O., Collura, T. F., Burgess, R. C., Morris, H. H., Hamano, T. et al. (1995a) "Subdural potentials at orbitofrontal and mesial prefrontal areas accompanying anticipation and decision making in humans: a comparison with Bereitschaftspotentials," *Electroencephalography and Clinical Neurophysiology*, 95(3): 206–212.

Ikeda, A., Luders, H. O., Shibasaki, H., Collura, T. F., Burgess, R. C., Morris, H. H. et al. (1995b) "Movement-related potentials associated with bilateral simultaneous and unilateral movements recorded from human supplementary motor area," *Electroencephalography and Clinical Neurophysiology*, 95(5): 323–334.

Jasper, H. H. (1936) "Cortical excitatory state and synchronism in the control of bioelectric autonomous rhythms," *Cold Spring Harbor Symposia in Quantitative Biology*, 4: 32–338.

Joffe, D. (1992) *Lexicor NRS-24 BioLex Operator's Manual*, Boulder, CO: Lexicor Corp.

John, E. R. (2001) "A field theory of consciousness," *Consciousness and Cognition*, 10: 184–213.

John, E. R. (2002) "The neurophysics of consciousness," *Brain Research Reviews*, 39: 1–28.

John, E. R. (2005) "From synchronous neuronal discharges to subjective awareness?" *Progress in Brain Research*, 150: 143–171.

Jung, R. (1939) "Das Elektroencephalogram und seine klinische Anwendung" ("The electroencephalogram and its clinical application"), *Nervenarzt*, 12: 569–591.

Kaiser, D. A. (1994) "QEEG: methodological issues," *Interest in Films as Measured by Subjective and Behavioral Ratings and Topographic EEG*, University of California, Los Angeles, retrieved May 27, 2013 from: www.skiltopo.com/papers/applied/articles/dakdiss2.htm.

Kaiser, D. A. (2008) Personal communication.

Kaiser, D. A. (2010) "Brodmann montage," retrieved May 27, 2013 from: www.skiltopo.com/papers/BrodmannMontageKaiser-v2.pdf.

Kim, J. (Ed.) (1993) *Supervenience and Mind: Selected Philosophical Essays*, Cambridge: Cambridge University Press.

Kinney, J. A. S., McKay, C. L, Mensch, A. J., and Luria, S. M. (1973) "Visual evoked responses elicited by rapid stimulation," *Electroencephalography and Clinical Neurophysiology*, 34: 7–13.

Kroger, W. S. and Schneider, S. A. (1959) "An electronic aid for hypnotic induction: a preliminary report," *International Journal of Clinical and Experimental Hypnosis*, 7: 93–98.

Kropotov, J. D. (2009) *Quantitative EEG, Event-Related Potentials, and Neurotherapy*, Amsterdam: Elsevier.

Larsen, S. (2006) *The Healing Power of Neurofeedback*, Rochester, VT: Healing Arts Press.

Larsen, S. (2012) *The Neurofeedback Solution*, Rochester, VT: Healing Arts Press.

Lee, K., Schottler, F., Oliver, M., and Lynch, G. (1980) "Brief bursts of high-frequency stimulation produce two types of structural change in rat hippocampus," *Journal of Neurophysiology*, 44(2): 247–258.

Lewerenz, C. (1963) "A factual report on the brain wave synchronizer," *Hypnosis Quarterly*, 6(4): 23.

Linden, M., Gevirtz, R., Isenhart, R., and Fisher, T. (1996) "Event related potentials of subgroups of children with attention deficit hyperactivity disorder and the implications for EEG biofeedback," *Journal of Neurotherapy*, Spring/Summer: 22–31.

Lubar, J. F. (1991) "Discourse on the development of EEG diagnostics and biofeedback for attention-deficit/hyperactivity disorders," *Biofeedback and Self-Regulation*, 16(3): 201–225.

Lubar, J. F. (1997) "Neocortical dynamics: implications for understanding the role of neurofeedback and related techniques for the enhancement of attention," *Applied Psychophysiology and Biofeedback*, 22: 111–126.

Lubar, J. F. (1998a) "An evaluation of the short-term and long-term effects of AVS (sound and light) on QEEG: surprising findings," presented at the 1998 Winter Brain Meeting, Palm Springs, CA.

Lubar, J. F. (1998b) "The effects of single session and multi-session audio-visual stimulation (AVS) at dominant alpha frequency and two times dominant alpha frequency on cortical EEG," *Journal of Neurotherapy*, 2(3): 66–67.

Lubar, J. (2003) "Neurofeedback for the management of attention deficit disorders," in M. S. Schwartz and F. Andrasik (Eds.) *Biofeedback: A Practitioner's Guide*, New York and London: Guilford Press, pp. 409–437.

Lubar, J., Congedo, M., and Askew, J. H. (2003) "Low resolution electromagnetic tomography (LORETA) of cerebral activity in chronic depressive disorder," *International Journal of Psychophysiology*, 49(3): 175–185.

Lubar, J. F., Swartwood, M. O., Swartwood, J. N., and O'Donnell, P. H. (1995) "Evaluation of the effectiveness of EEG neurofeedback training for ADHD in a clinical setting as measured by changes in TOVA scores, behavioral ratings, and WISC-R performance," *Applied Psychophysiology and Biofeedback*, 20(1): 83–99.

Lueders, H., Bustamante, L. A., Zablow, L., and Goldensohn, E. S. (1981) "The independence of closely spaced discrete experimental spike foci," *Neurology*, 31(7): 846–851.

Lutz, A., Greischar, L. L., Rawlings, N. V., Ricard, M., and Davidson, R. J. (2004) "Long-term meditators self-induce high-amplitude gamma synchrony during mental practice," *Proceedings of the National Academy of Sciences*, 101(46): 16369–16373.

McGillem, C. D. and Aunon, J. I. (1977) "Measurements of signal components in single visually evoked brain potentials," *IEEE Transactions on Biomedical Engineering*, 24(3): 232–241.

McNight, J. T. and Fehmi, L. G. (2001) "Attention and neurofeedback synchrony training: clinical results and their significance," *Journal of Neurotherapy*, 5(1).

Makeig, S., Debener, S., Onton, J., and Delorme, A. (2004) "Mining event-related brain dynamics," *Trends in Cognitive Sciences*, 8(5): 204–210.

Manns, A., Miralles, R., and Adrian, H. (1981) "The application of audiostimulation and electromyographic biofeedback to bruxism and myofascial pain-dysfunction syndrome," *Oral Surgery*, 52(3): 247–252.

Maust, D. (1997) "Feedback made simple," 5th Annual Winter Conference on Brain Function/EEG, February 21–25, Palm Springs, CA.

Maust, D. (1999) "Wideband amplitude reduction: why it ought to be in your bag of tricks and when you should be careful with it," *Proceedings of the Winter Brain Conference*, Palm Springs, CA.

Mentis, M., Alexander, G., Grady, C., Krasuski, J., Pietrini, P., Strassburger, T., et al. (1997) "Frequency variation of a pattern-flash visual stimulus during PET differentially activates brain from striate through frontal cortex," *Neuroimage*, 5: 116–128.

Miller, N. E. (1967) "Laws of learning relevant to its biological basis," *Proceedings of the American Philosophical Society*, 111: 315–325.

Miller, N. E. (1969) "Learning of visceral and glandular responses," *Science*, 163: 434–445.

Millman J. and Halkias, C. C. (1972) *Integrated Electronics: Analog and Digital Circuits and Systems*, New York: McGraw-Hill.

Monastra, V. J. (2005) "Electroencephalographic biofeedback (neurotherapy) as a treatment for attention deficit hyperactivity disorder: rationale and empirical foundation," in L. M. Hirschberg, S. Chiu, and J. A. Frazier (Eds.) *Child and Adolescent Psychiatric Clinics of North America*, 14(1): 55–82.

Monastra, V. J., Lynn, S., Linden, M., Lubar, J., Gruzelier, J., and LaVaque, T. (2005) "Electroencephalographic biofeedback in the treatment of attention-deficit/ hyperactivity disorder," *Applied Psychophysiology and Biofeedback*, 30(2): 95–114.

Moss, D. (2004) "Heart rate variability (HRV) biofeedback," *Psychophysiology Today*, 1: 4–11.

Mulert, C., Jager, L., Schmitt, R., Bussfeld, P., Pogarell, O., Joller, H., et al. (2004) "Integration of fMRI and simultaneous EEG: towards a comprehensive understanding of localization and time-course of brain activity in target detection," *Neuroimage*, 22: 83–94.

Naatanen, R. (1975) "Selective attention and evoked potentials in humans—a critical review," *Biological Psychology*, 2: 237–307.

Nash, J. F. (1950) "Equilibrium points in n-person games," *Proceedings of the National Academy of Sciences*, 36: 48–49.

Neidermeyer, E. and Lopes da Silva, F. H. (2005) *Electroencephalography: Basic Principles, Clinical Applications, and Related Fields*, Phildelphia, PA: Lippincott Williams & Wilkins.

Nunez, P. L. (1995) "Toward a physics of neocortex," in P. L. Nunez (Ed.) *Neocortical Dynamics and Human EEG Rhythms*, New York: Oxford University Press, pp. 68–132.

Nunez, P. L. (2000) "Toward a quantitative description of large scale neocortical dynamic function and EEG," *Behavioral and Brain Sciences*, 5(8): 371–398.

Nunez, P. L. and Pilgreen, K. L. (1991) "The spline-laplacian in clinical neurophysiology: a method to improve EEG spatial resolution," *Journal of Clinical Neurophysiology*, 8(4): 397–413.

Ochs, L. (2006) "The low energy neurofeedback system (LENS): theory, background, and introduction," *Journal of Neurotherapy*, 10(2–3): 5–39.

Oppenheim, A. V. and Shafer, R. W. (1975) *Digital Signal Processing*, Englewood Cliffs, NJ: Prentice Hall.

Othmer, S. (2010) "Introduction to infra-low frequency training," retrieved May 27, 2013 from www.eeginfo.com/newsletter/?p=523.

Othmer, S. and Othmer, S. F. (2008) "Infra-low frequency training," retrieved May 27, 2013 from www.eeginfo.com/research/articles/Infra-LowFrequencyTraining.pdf.

Pascual-Marqui, R. D. (1999) "Review of methods for solving the EEG inverse problem," *International Journal of Bioelectromagnetism*, 1(1): 75–86.

Pascual-Marqui, R. D. (2002) "Standardized low resolution brain electromagnetic tomography (sLORETA): technical details," *Methods and Findings in Experimental and Clinical Pharmacology*, 24: 5–12.

Pascual-Marqui, R. D. (2011) "The human brain resting state networks based on high time resolution EEG: comparison to metabolism-based networks," *Proceedings of the Annual Meeting of the International Society for Neurofeedback and Research*, Keynote presentation, retrieved May 27, 2013 from www.isnr.org.

Pascual-Marqui, R. D., Michel, C. M, and Lehmann, D. (1994) "Low resolution electromagnetic tomography: a new method for localizing electrical activity in the brain," *International Journal of Psychophysiology*, 18: 49–65.

Patrick. G. J. (1996) "Improved neuronal regulation in ADHD: an application of fifteen sessions of photic-driven EEG neurotherapy," *Journal of Neurotherapy*, 1(4): 27–36.

Peniston, E. and Kulkosky, P. (1989) "Alpha-theta brainwave training and beta-endorphin levels in alcoholics," *Alcoholism: Clinical and Experimental Research*, 13(2): 271–279.

Peniston, E. and Kulkosky, P. (1990) "Alcoholic personality and alpha-theta brainwave training," *Medical Psychotherapy*, 3: 37–55.

Peniston, E., Marrinan, D., Deming, W., and Kulkosky, P. (1993) "EEG alpha-theta brainwave synchronization in Vietnam theatre veterans with combat-related post-traumatic stress disorder and alcohol abuse," *Advances in Medical Psychotherapy*, 6: 37–49.

Pieron, H. (1982) "Melanges dedicated to Monsieur Pierre Janet," *Acta Psychiatrica Belgica*, 1: 7–112.

Price, J. and Budzynski, T. (2008) "Anxiety, EEG patterns and neurofeedback," in T. Budzynski, H. Budzynski, J. E. Evans, and A. Abarbanal (Eds.) *Introduction to Quantitative EEG and Neurofeedback* (2nd ed.), Amsterdam: Elsevier, pp. 337–364.

Plotkin, W. B. and Rice, K. M. (1981) "Biofeedback as a placebo: anxiety reduction facilitated by training in either suppression or enhancement of alpha brainwaves," *Journal of Consulting and Clinical Psychology*, 49(4): 590.

Prichep, L., John, E., Ferris, S., Reisberg, B., Almas, M., Alper, K., et al. (1994) "Quantitative EEG correlates of cognitive deterioration in the elderly," *Neurobiology of Aging*, 15(1): 85–90.

Regan, D. (1966) "Some characteristics of average steady-state and transient responses evoked by modulated light," *Electroencephalography and Clinical Neurophysiology*, 20: 238–248.

Regan, D. (1989) *Human Brain Electrophysiology*, New York: Elsevier.

Rizzuto, D. S., Madsen, J. R., Bromfield, E. B., Schulze-Bonhage, A., Seelig, D., Aschenbrenner-Scheive, R., et al. (2003) "Reset of human neocortical oscillations during a working memory task," *Proceedings of the National Academy of Sciences*, 100(13): 7931–7936.

Robbins, J. (2001) "The mental edge," *Outside Magazine*, 26(4): 131–134.

Rockstroh, B., Elbert, T., Canavan, A., Lutzenberger, W., and N. Birbaumer (1989) *Slow Cortical Potentials and Behavior*, Baltimore, MD: Urban & Schwarzenberg.

Ros, T., Bloom, P., Benjamin, L., Moseley, M., and Gruzelier, J. (2006) "Neurofeedback peak performance training in microsurgery: a controlled study," Society for Applied Neuroscience, Swansea, September 2006.

Rosenfeld, J. P., Stamm, J., Elbert, T., Rockstroh, B., Birbaumer, N., and Roger, M. (1984) "Biofeedback of event related potentials," in R. Karrer, J. Cohen, and P. Tueting (Eds.) *Brain and Information: Event-Related Potentials: Annals of the New York Academy of Sciences*, 425: 653–666.

Rosenfeld, P. (1997) "EEG biofeedback of frontal alpha asymmetry in affective disorders," *Biofeedback*, 25(1): 8–12.

Rossiter, T. R. (2004) "The effectiveness of neurofeedback and stimulant drugs in treating AD/HD: Part I. Review of methodological issues," *Applied Psychophysiology and Biofeedback*, 29(2): 135–140.

Rossiter, T. R. (2005) "The effectiveness of neurofeedback and stimulant drugs in treating AD/HD: Part II. Replication," *Applied Psychophysiology and Biofeedback*, 29(4): 233–243.

Rossiter, T. R. and La Vaque, T. J. (1995) "A comparison of EEG biofeedback and psychostimulants in treating attention deficit/hyperactivity disorders," *Journal of Neurotherapy*, 1: 48–59.

Rubin, E., Sakiem, H., Nobler, M., and Moeller, J. (1994) "Brain imaging studies of antidepressant treatments," *Psychiatric Annals*, 24(12): 653–658.

Russell, H. (1996) "Entrainment combined with multimodal rehabilitation of a 43-year-old severely impaired postaneurysm patient," *Biofeedback and Self Regulation*, 21(4).

Russell, H., Collura, T. F., and Frederick, J. (2007) "The possible use of inexpensive sensory stimulation technologies to improve IQ test scores and behavior," *Proceedings of the 2nd Symposium on Music, Rhythm, and the Brain*, Stanford University, Stanford, CA.

Rutter, P. J. (2011) Personal communication.

Sabado, S. M. (1970) *Basic Principles of Operant Conditioning*, retrieved May 27, 2013 from www.scribd.com/doc/28687783/Basic-Principles-of-Operant-Conditioning

Saltzberg, B. (1976) "A model for relating ripples in the EEG power spectral density to transient patterns of brain electrical activity induced by subcortical spiking," *IEEE Transactions on Biomedical Engineering*, 23(4): 355–356.

Sappey-Marinier, D., Calabrese, G., Fein, G., Hugg, J., Biggins, C., and Weiner, M. (1992) "Effect of photic stimulation on human visual cortex lactate and phosphates using 1H and 31P magnetic resonance spectroscopy," *Journal of Cerebral Blood Flow and Metabolism*, 12(4): 584–592.

Sarnthein, J., Petsche, H., Rappelsberger, P., Shaw, G. L., and von Stein, A. (1998) "Synchronization between prefrontal and posterior association cortex during human working memory," *Proceedings of the National Academy of Sciences*, 95: 7092–7096.

Sato, K., Kitajima, H., Mimura, K., Hirota, H., Tagawa, Y., and Ochi, N. (1971) "Cerebral visual evoked potentials in relation to EEG," *Electroencephalography and Clinical Neurophysiology*, 30: 123–138.

Schack, B. and Klimesch, W. (2002) "Frequency characteristics of evoked and oscillatory electroencephalographic activity in a human memory scanning task," *Neuroscience Letters*, 331: 107–110.

Schack, B., Vath, N., Hetsche, H., Geissler, H. G., and Moller, E. (2002) "Phase-coupling of theta-gamma EEG rhythms during short-term memory processing," *International Journal of Psychophysiology*, 44(2): 143–163.

Schechter, G. and Buchsbaum, M. (1973) "The effects of attention, stimulus intensity, and individual differences on the average evoked response," *Psychophysiology*, 10(4): 392–400.

Scott, W. and Kaiser, D. (1998) "Augmenting chemical dependency treatment with neurofeedback training," *Journal of Neurotherapy*, 3(1): 66.

Scott, W., Kaiser, D., Othmer, S., and Sideroff, S. (2005) "Effects of an EEG biofeedback protocol on a mixed substance abusing population," *The American Journal of Drug and Alcohol Abuse*, 31: 455–469.

Sekihara, K., Sahani, M., and Nagarajan, S. (2005) "Localization bias and spatial resolution of adaptive and non-adaptive spatial filters for MEG source reconstruction," *NeuroImage*, 25: 1056–1067.

Sethi, R. (2007) "Nash equilibrium," in *International Encyclopedia of Social Sciences* (2nd ed.), pp. 540–542, retrieved May 27, 2013 from: www.columbia.edu/~rs328/NashEquilibrium.pdf.

Shaw, J. C. (2003) *The Brain's Alpha Rhythms and the Mind*, New York: Elsevier.

Siever, D. (1997a) "The effectiveness of white light and sound pulsed stimulation as applied to chronic pain," 5th Annual Winter Conference on Brain Function/EEG Modifications and Training, Advanced Meeting/Colloquium, Palm Springs, CA.

Siever, D. (1997b) *The Rediscovery of Audio-Visual Entrainment Technology*, Edmonton, Alberta: Comptronic Devices Limited.

Silberstein, R. B. (1990) "Electroencephalographic attention monitor," US Patent Number 4955388.

Silberstein, R. B. (1994) "Equipment for testing or measuring brain activity," US Patent Number 5331969.

Silberstein, R. B. (1995) "Steady-state visually evoked potentials, brain resonances, and cognitive processes," in P. L. Nunez (Ed.) *Neocortical Dynamics and Human EEG Rhythms*, New York, Oxford University Press, pp. 272–303.

Silberstein, R. B. (2006) "Dynamic sculpting of brain functional connectivity and mental rotation aptitude," *Progress in Brain Research*, 159: 63–76.

Silberstein, R. B., Schier, M. A., Pipingas, A., Ciorciari, J., Wood, S. R., and Simpson, D. G. (1990) "Steady-state visually evoked potential topography associated with a visual vigilance task," *Brain Topography*, 3(2): 337–347.

Singer, K. (2004) "The effect of neurofeedback on performance anxiety in dancers," presented at the 14th Annual Meeting of the International Association for Dance Medicine and Science, San Francisco, CA, October 15–17, *Journal of Dance Medicine and Science*, 8(3): 78–81.

Skarda, C. A. and Freeman, W. J. (1987) "How brains make chaos in order to make sense of the world," *Behavioral and Brain Sciences*, 10: 161–195.

Skinner, B. F. (1938) *The Behavior of Organisms: An Experimental Analysis*, New York: Appleton-Century.

Skinner, B. F. (1948) "Superstition in the pigeon," *Journal of Experimental Psychology*, 38: 168–172, retrieved May 27, 2013 from: http://psychclassics.yorku.ca/Skinner/Pigeon/.

Skinner, B. F. (1956) "A case history in scientific method," *American Psychologist*, 11: 221–233. Also published in S. Koch (1958) *Psychology: A Study of a Science*, vol. II, New York: McGraw-Hill.

Smith, M. (2011) "Infra-low frequency: A proposed mechanism," retrieved May 27, 2013 from: www.bec-eeg.com/ilf-proposed-mechanism.pdf.

Sokhadze, T. M., Cannon, R. L., and Trudeau, D. L. (2008) "EEG biofeedback as a treatment for substance abuse disorders: review, rating of efficacy, and recommendations for further research," *Applied Psychophysiology and Biofeedback*, 33: 1–28.

Spong, P., Haider, M., and Lindsley, D. B. (1969) "Selective attentiveness and cortical evoked responses to visual and auditory stimuli," in R. Haber (Ed.) *Information Processing Approaches to Visual Perception*, New York: Holt, Rinehart & Winston, pp. 398–401.

Srinivarsan, T. M. (1988) "Nonvolitional biofeedback as a therapy," in T. M. Srinivarsan (Ed.) *Energy Medicine Around the World*, Phoenix, AZ: Gabriel Press, pp. 157–166.

Stahl, C. and Collura, T. F. (2012) "Assessing the effects of subthreshold magnetic stimulation on brain activation using sLORETA," *NeuroConnections*, Winter: 34–36.

Starr, C. and Taggart, R. (2003) *The Unity and Diversity of Life* (10th ed.), Mason, OH: Cengagebrain.com.

Sterman, B. (2008) Speech delivered at the Claude Bernard Society Meeting, Annual Meeting of the Association for Applied Psychophysiology and Biofeedback.

Sterman, M. B. (1996) "Physiological origins and functional correlates of EEG rhythmic activities: implications for self-regulation," *Biofeedback and Self-Regulation*, 21(1): 3–33.

Sterman, M. B. (2000) "Basic concepts and clinical findings in the treatment of seizure disorders with EEG operant conditioning," *Clinical Electroencephalography and Neuroscience*, 31(1): 45–55.

Sterman, M. B. and Kaiser, D. A. (2001) "Comodulation: a new QEEG analysis metric for assessment of structural and functional disorders of the CNS," *Journal of Neurotherapy*, 4: 73–84.

Sterman, M. B., Mann, C. A., Kaiser, D. A., and Suyenobu, B. Y. (1994) "Multiband topographic EEG analysis of a simulated visuomoter aviation task," *International Journal of Psychophysiology*, 16: 49–56.

Stoller, L. (2011) "Z-scores, combinatorics, and phase transitions," *Journal of Neurotherapy*, 15(1): 35–53.

Suzuki, A. and Kirino, E. (2004) "Combined LORETA and fMRI study of recognition of eyes and eye movement in schizophrenia," *Elsevier International Congress Series*, 1270: 348–351.

Thatcher, R. W. (1997) "Neural coherence and the content of consciousness," *Consciousness and Cognition*, 6: 42–49.

Thatcher, R. W. (1998) "A predator-prey model of human cerebral development," in K. Newell and P. Molenar (Eds.) *Applications of Nonlinear Dynamics to Developmental Process Modeling*, Mahwah, NJ: Lawrence Erlbaum Associates, pp. 87–128.

Thatcher, R. W. (1998) "EEG normative databases and EEG biofeedback," *Journal of Neurotherapy*, 2(4): 8–39.

Thatcher, R. W. (1999) "EEG database guided neurotherapy," in J. R. Evans and A. Abarbanel (Eds.) *Introduction to Quantitative EEG and Neurofeedback*, San Diego, CA: Academic Press.

Thatcher, R. W. (2000) "EEG operant conditioning (biofeedback) and traumatic brain injury," *Clinical EEG*, 31(1): 38–44.

Thatcher, R. W. (2007) *Hand Calculations of EEG Coherence, Phase Delays and Brain Connectivity*, St. Petersburg: Applied Neurosciences.

Thatcher, R. W. (2008) "Z-score EEG biofeedback: conceptual foundations," *Neuro-Connections*, April 2008.

Thatcher, R. W. and Lubar, J. F. (2009) "History of the scientific standards of QEEG normative databases," in T. Budzynski, H. Budzynski, J. Evans, and D. Abarbanel (Eds.) *QEEG and Neurofeedback* (2nd ed.), Amsterdam: Elsevier, pp. 29–59.

Thatcher, R. W., Krause, P. J., and Hrybyk, M. (1986) "Cortico-cortical associations and EEG coherence: a two-compartmental model," *Electroencephalography and Clinical Neurophysiology*, 64: 123–143.

Thatcher, R. W., Walker, R. A., and Guidice, S. (1987) "Human cerebral hemispheres develop at different rates and ages," *Science*, 236: 1110–1113.

Thatcher, R. W., North, D., and Biver, C. (2005) "EEG and intelligence: univariate and multivariate comparisons between EEG coherence, EEG phase delay and power," *Clinical Neurophysiology*, 116(9): 2129–2141.

Thatcher, R. W., North, D., and Biver, C. (2005) "EEG inverse solutions and parametric vs. non-parametric statistics of low resolution electromagnetic tomography (LORETA)," *Clinical EEG and Neuroscience*, 36(1): 1–9.

Thatcher, R. W., North, D., and Biver, C. (2005) "Evaluation and validity of a LORETA normative EEG database," *Clinical EEG and Neuroscience*, 36(2): 116–122.

Thatcher, R. W., North, D., and Biver, C. (2005) "EEG and intelligence: relations between EEG coherence, EEG phase delay and power," *Clinical Neurophysiology*, 116: 2129–2141.

Thatcher, R. W., Biver, C. J., and North, D. (2006) "Spatio-temporal current course correlations and cortical connectivity," EEG and Clinical Neuroscience Society Annual Meeting, Boston, MA, *EEG and Clinical EEG and Neuroscience*, (37)2: 279–300.

Thatcher, R. W., Walker, R. A., Biver, C., North, D., and Curtin, R. (2003) "Quantitative EEG normative databases: validation and clinical correlation," *Journal of Neurotherapy*, 7: 87–122.

Thompson, L. and Thompson, M. (2008a) "QEEG and neurofeedback for assessment and effective intervention with attention deficit hyperactivity disorder (ADHD)," in T. Budzynski, H. Budzynski, J. E. Evans, and A. Abarbanal (Eds.) *Introduction to Quantitative EEG and Neurofeedback* (2nd ed.), Amsterdam: Elsevier, pp. 337–364.

Thompson, L. and Thompson, M. (2008b) "Asperger's syndrome intervention: combining neurofeedback, biofeedback and metacognition," in T. Budzynski, H. Budzynski, J. E. Evans, and A. Abarbanal (Eds.) *Introduction to Quantitative EEG and Neurofeedback* (2nd ed.), Amsterdam: Elsevier, pp. 337–364.

Thornton, K. (1999) "Exploratory investigation into mild brain injury and discriminant analysis with high frequency bands (32–64 Hz)," *Brain Injury*, August: 477–488.

Thornton, K. (2000) "Exploratory analysis: mild head injury, discriminant analysis with high frequency bands (32–64 Hz) under attentional activation conditions and does time heal?" *Journal of Neurotherapy*, 3: 1–10.

Thornton, K. and Carmody, D. (2009) "Eyes-closed and activation QEEG databases in predicting cognitive effectiveness and the inefficiency hypothesis, *Journal of Neurotherapy*, 13(1): 1–22.

Toman, J. (1941) "Flicker potentials and the alpha rhythm in man," *Journal of Neurophysiology*, 4: 51–61.

Townsend, R. (1973) "A device for generation and presentation of modulated light stimuli," *Electroencephalography and Clinical Neurophysiology*, 34, 97–99.

Townsend, R. E., Lubin, A., and Naitoh, P. (1975) "Stabilization of alpha frequency by sinusoidally modulated light," *Electroencephalography and Clinical Neurophysiology*, 39(5): 515–518.

Trudeau, D. L., Sokhadze, T. M., and Cannon, R. (2008) "Neurofeedback in alcohol and drug dependency," in T. Budzynski, H. Budzynski, J. E. Evans, and A. Abarbanal (Eds.) *Introduction to Quantitative EEG and Neurofeedback* (2nd ed.), Amsterdam: Elsevier, pp. 241–268.

Trudeau, D. L., Moore, J., Stockley, H., and Rubin, Y. (1999) "A pilot study of the effect of 18 Hz audio visual stimulation (AVS) on attention and concentration symptoms and on quantitative EEG (QEEG) in long term chronic fatigue," *Journal of Neurotherapy*, 4.

Van der Tweel, L. and Lunel, H. (1965) "Human visual responses to sinusoidally modulated light," *Electroencephalography and Clinical Neurophysiology*, 18: 587–598.

Van Hof, M. W. (1960) "The relation between the cortical responses to flash and to flicker in man," *Acta Physiologica Pharmacologica Neerlandica*, 9: 210–224.

Vitacco, D., Brandeis, D., Pascual-Marqui, R., and Martin, E. (2002) "Correspondence of event-related potential tomography and functional magnetic resonance imaging during language processing," *Human Brain Mapping*, 17: 4–12.

Von Stein, A. and Sarnthein, J. (2000) "Different frequencies for different scales of cortical integration: from local gamma to long range alpha/theta synchronization," *International Journal of Psychophysiology*, 38(3): 301–313.

Von Stein, A., Rappelsberger, P., Sarnthein, J., and Petsche, H. (1999) "Synchronization between temporal and parietal cortex during multimodal object processing in man," *Cerebral Cortex*, 9: 137–150.

Walker, J. E. (2011) "QEEG-guided neurofeedback for recurrent migraine headaches," *Clinical EEG and Neuroscience*, 42(1): 59–61.

Walker, J. E., Norman, C. A., and Weber, R. K. (2002) "Impact of qEEG-guided coherence training for patients with a mild closed head injury," *Journal of Neurotherapy*, 6(2): 31–43.

Walker, J. E., Kozlowski, G. P., and Lawson, R. (2007) "A modular activation/ coherence approach to evaluating clinical/QEEG correlations," *Journal of Neurotherapy*, 11(1): 25–44.

Walter, W. G. (1956) "Color illusions and aberrations during stimulation by flickering light," *Nature*, 177: 710.

Walter, W. G. and Walter, V. G. (1949) "The central effects of rhythmic sensory stimulation," *Electroencephalography and Clinical Neurophysiology*, 1, 57–86.

Watson, J. B. (1930) *Behaviorism* (revised ed.), Chicago, IL: University of Chicago Press.

Weiner, N. (1948) *Cybernetics: Or the Control and Communication in the Animal and the Machine*, New York: MIT Press, John Wiley & Sons.

Williams, J., Ramaswamy, D., and Oulhaj, A. (2006) "10 Hz flicker improves recognition memory in older people," *BMC Neuroscience*, 7(21): 1–7.

Wilson, J. (2001) "Adrenal fatigue: the 21st century stress syndrome," *Smart Publications*, Petaluma, CA.

Wu, J., Gillin, J., Buchsbaum, M., Hershey, T., Johnson, J., and Bunney, W. (1992) "Effect of sleep deprivation on brain metabolism of depressed patients," *American Journal of Psychiatry*, 149: 538–543.

Yemm, R. (1969) "Variations in the electrical activity of the human masseter muscle occuring in association with emotional stress," *Archives of Oral Biology*, 14: 873–878.

INDEX